Praise for C
Body, Revec

"Dr. Pentz, a thought leader in integrative mental health care, makes a compelling case for the relevance of an Ayurvedic practice that cleanses and rejuvenates body and soul. Combining ancient wisdom with stories from her own deeply personal journey toward healing, Dr. Pentz skillfully guides the reader through an immersive eight-day program of cleansing, meditation, and massage that will enhance physical, emotional, and spiritual well-being. Strongly recommended."

—James Lake, MD, integrative psychiatrist and the author of ten short books on alternative and integrative treatments of mental health problems

"Judith is a wise kindred spirit who will take you on a journey to your most grounded, most spiritually aware self. This book has all the science and all the soul you'll need to restore a sustainable sense of self-care in your life."

—Joan Borysenko, PhD, *NY Times* bestselling author of *Minding the Body, Mending the Mind*

"Judith Pentz combines a marvelous mix of modern and ancient wellness wisdom in her book that will bring readers much peace, calm, and healing."

—KJ Landis, author of *Happy Healthy You*

"Dr. Judith Pentz is a connoisseur of techniques and therapies that have been proven to work over millennia in other cultures. A key example is panchakarma, drawn from the Ayurveda healing tradition of ancient India. In *Cleanse Your Body, Reveal Your Soul*, Dr. Pentz reveals how and why this healing approach has endured over centuries and how it can benefit those of us in modern cultures as well. If you have an instinctive reluctance toward mind-bending medications, this subtle, gentle way of healing your body-mind deserves your attention."

—Larry Dossey, MD, author of *One Mind: How Our Individual Mind Is Part of a Greater Consciousness and Why It Matters*

"In *Cleanse Your Body, Reveal Your Soul* Judith Pentz, MD, provides us with an Ayurvedic roadmap to health, illuminated by years of personal exploration as a physician and healer. A comprehensive guide to the practices and process of Ayurvedic medicine, Pentz peppers this compendium of wisdom with explanations of herbal recipes, foods, medicinal preparations, and yogic practices. Pentz walks with us as a wise guide, so that we may understand and enact these methods in our daily lives, reminding us always that the journey to health and balance is as much a spiritual unfolding, as it is physically rejuvenating."

—Leslie Korn, PhD, MPH, author of *Nutrition Essentials for Mental Health: A Complete Guide to the Food-Mood Connection*

"*Cleanse Your Body, Reveal Your Soul* is a powerful retelling of Dr. Pentz's personal journey, one that will resonate with readers who seek health through balance, balance through health, and inspiration for action from an accomplished modern-day healer."

—James Greenblatt, MD, chief medical officer/VP of medical services at Walden Behavioral Care

"A dazzling and radiant book with a message straight from the Goddess. *Cleanse Your Body, Reveal Your Soul* addresses how to heal from chronic, pain, illness, trauma, and PTSD. Most of us have some form of one of these common imbalances that Western medicine often falls short of addressing. Adverse experiences can entangle us and Ayurveda offers simplicity as the antidote. Dr. Judith Eve Pentz's compelling account of her own Pancha Karma journey reveals why the healing wisdom of Ayurveda in its gorgeous and essential nature is still as relevant today as it was four thousand years ago."

—Elise Marie Collins, author of *Super Ager: You Can Look Younger, Have More Energy, a Better Memory, and Live a Long and Healthy Life*

CLEANSE
your body,
REVEAL
your soul

CLEANSE
your body,
REVEAL
your soul

SUSTAINABLE WELL-BEING THROUGH THE ANCIENT POWER OF AYURVEDA PANCHAKARMA THERAPY

Judith Eve Pentz, MD

WISDOM TEACHER, SAGE, & ALCHEMIST

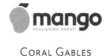

mango
PUBLISHING GROUP

CORAL GABLES

Published by Mango Publishing Group, a division of Mango Media Inc.

Cover Illustration: © Vasiliy Soldatov/shutterstock.com
Cover Design, Layout & Design: Morgane Leoni

For permission requests, please contact the publisher at:
Mango Publishing Group
2850 S Douglas Road, 2nd Floor
Coral Gables, FL 33134 USA
info@mango.bz

For special orders, quantity sales, course adoptions and corporate sales, please email the publisher at sales@mango.bz. For trade and wholesale sales, please contact Ingram Publisher Services at customer.service@ingramcontent.com or +1.800.509.4887.

Cleanse Your Body, Reveal Your Soul: Sustainable Well-Being Through the Ancient Power of Ayurveda Panchakarma Therapy

Library of Congress Cataloging-in-Publication number: 2020940889
ISBN: (print) 978-1-64250-378-4, (ebook) 978-1-64250-379-1
BISAC: OCC011000—BODY, MIND & SPIRIT / Healing / General

Printed in the United States of America

Wisdom says that I am nothing.
Love says that I am everything.
Instead of searching for what you do not have,
find out what it is you never lost.
If you change yourself,
you will find that no other change is needed.

—Sri Nisargadatta Maharaj

Contents

Invitation to
the Reader

Too many of us have tried just about everything to heal emotional wounds and shift them so they are no longer obstacles to happiness. It's baffling. If we are actively seeking to change, then why don't we heal? What if I told you that making a few small changes can make a dramatic, life-altering difference?

What if I told you that you could find healing on the cellular level, so the shifts are long-lasting and transformative?

The magic word: Ayurveda.

It means the knowledge of life. And one little ayurvedic practice—panchakarma—makes all the difference. Panchakarma can be described as a fivefold detoxification treatment involving massage, herbal therapy, and other procedures. Let me paint a picture of some of panchakarma's simple life-giving methods: Imagine massages with warm sesame oil that soothe. The warmed oil, gently poured on your forehead, which can bliss you out. Nurturing food served to support your process. These methods have a component beneath them that is reverent of the knowledge of life. The foundation of panchakarma is tender, loving care of our body, mind, and soul, something we are short on in these times. Yet the results are not merely temporarily palliative. The methods guide you to find calm so you may come home to your essence. That is what lasts.

All of my life, I have sought a way to return to the soul. I believe this to be possible for my clients, in my work as an integrative psychiatrist, and I believe this for myself. Yet, so often I see people slip into their old ways of pain, even when they desire to move forward. I've always sought a way to create change in a sustainable way. I've always known there must be a way to unlearn the pain that creates a chronic pattern in the mind and keeps the body a container for the old pain. For a long time, I saw myself and others experience temporary relief or incremental shifts. But I always wondered: is there something deeper that, if I could tap into it, would shift me in such a profound way that I could be changed from the inside out? And from which place, the unfolding come with ease and joy?

I have found it.

My search has been long, but not without happiness. My search has been difficult, and it took courage. But now I experience a world of greater contentment and infinite possibilities. I feel cleansed and renewed from the inside, in a way that has rejuvenated my spirit and returned me to soul freedom.

Panchakarma: it touches every cell of your being. Throughout this book, I weave the narrative of my transformative experience with panchakarma on a trip to India, but provide tools and techniques that you can utilize at home. In each chapter, you will learn more about these tools and how to use them. All of them will help support you on your journey to wholeness. These techniques are best used before having a panchakarma experience. I did this way and found it to be most helpful. For instance, I know that simply doing *shirodhara* (slow release of warmed sesame oil on your third eye) once a month creates an incredible sense of calm and bliss that can last for days.

How have I changed, you might ask? I have a deeper awareness of who I am in the essence of my being. Patterns or habits that I once perceived as obstacles, or did not even know were part of me, have fallen by the wayside. Bringing beauty into my life is most important. Now I walk in the wonder and beauty of life, and I know that at the deepest level, I am changed. I have the capacity to be an observer of the day I am entering, so that I am present with its challenges in a more balanced way. When I encounter people who are less than kind, I can now interact and not take their behavior personally. My level of discernment has grown immensely. I know when to separate myself from a toxic space by taking a quick walk outdoors to reconnect with nature. These quick walks aid my perspective as I hear the birds sing and feel the sun's warmth on my skin. Then I return. In the past, I found myself triggered in countless ways and found that, come evening, I could not recover from the demands of the day. With the aid of my self-care practices and daily ayurvedic rituals, I can maintain my capacity to be present long after the immediate effects of panchakarma.

That's the power of panchakarma, and it's the reason I halted my integrative psychiatry practice for five weeks so that I could take a trip to Nagpur, India, in spring 2014. In fall 2013, I yearned to go into retreat. I needed to shift how I was approaching my life and my work with those in my practice. I felt a strong internal push to be more authentic and present with parts of my being that have been tamped down by all my years of being a more allopathic-trained psychiatrist (a model based on human-made, scientific remedies). At the same time that I needed to be authentic, I also wanted the people who presented themselves to me to be authentic. Yet, I pondered, how would that manifest in the current paradigm in which I have been working? The answer was so complicated that I couldn't get to it with words. Instead, I found it in images. I have a deck of Zen cards created by Osho Zen, and one of the cards depicts a being breaking through a wall and standing empowered. I saw myself in that picture but I still felt reluctant to move in that direction. How could I do that while maintaining an active practice that operated under a certain allopathic model?

That fall, I had been in the Esalen Institute in Big Sur, California, for a retreat. I joined others who were also seeking healthier ways to support people going through an emotional breakthrough—something that can be seen as a psychotic break in the current paradigm under which I then worked. Yet many of these amazing people with whom I shared this healing space had experiences that constituted a move beyond the need to be on medication, thriving in many ways. While at Esalen, we had time to receive nurturing massages and soak in the hot tubs by the sea. We were served healing food that often was harvested from the land on which we walked. We participated in healing sessions with intuitives working on site. During one of these sessions I made a request—a divine declaration. I asked for the time and space to be able to share what was in my heart and share it with groups in healing places like Esalen. It was from here the idea was born to create time and space for myself. From here, I decided to go to Nagpur.

Awakening

Who does this? Who puts a life on hold, a life that appears successful from most any perspective, to trek to distant Nagpur and then to the southern Himalayas? In truth, the inner urge to go to India was born about ten years ago, when I sought out an ayurvedic physician, Sunil Joshi, MD (Ayu), in Albuquerque for my first panchakarma. Joshi had moved to New Mexico more than twenty years ago from Nagpur and began to offer panchakarma only to those who were interested. He is clinically trained as a medical doctor from India and has a master's degree in Ayurveda with a focus on panchakarma. He has developed clinics in Albuquerque and Nagpur specifically for panchakarma treatment, and divides his time between these clinics throughout the year. He also travels to Europe to do consultations.

As with all meaningful journeys, my story begins with an awakening—of a part of myself that had been asleep. Even with previous experience in panchakarma, I was not expecting what came. As I explored what happened to me, I realized that I was not alone—yet no one had ever mentioned this wondrous opening as part of the cleanse. I was curious about this. I felt the need to share my personal journey so others could know what is possible in this lifetime. It is a way to touch the part of the Divine within, yet there are all these other benefits for one's physical, emotional, and mental health.

But let us start at the beginning, or what I think might be the beginning, of my opening up to more possibilities. I live near an *acequia* (a community-operated watercourse) in Albuquerque, New Mexico, and I often walk there. One day, after the final day of my fourth panchakarma (PK) experience in 2011, as I was walking, I saw magic, light, and wonder everywhere. The light of that day had a luminescence I had rarely experienced. Sunlight danced on the water. Horsetails appeared brighter green with a white aura around them. Tall grass growing on the side of the acequia shifted in the wind. Dragonflies shimmered as they floated over the water. Rustling cottonwood leaves added to the symphony of sound. A dove called in the distance. I was present and aware. I was in awe. Listening to the water spilling over the dam created even more peace within.

As I contemplated all that was shifting within my being, I was increasingly aware of emotional patterns in my second and third chakras. Weighing heavily on my heart were issues about family and tribe. My soul was searching for answers about setting healthy boundaries. In that moment, insight flooded me.

How was such a breakthrough possible? For a long time, I had explored and continue to explore different therapy routes to move emotional obstacles and wounds. I had seen some movement, even resolution, of some issues, yet I wasn't completely satisfied. Yet here was a modality that had been touted for its physical benefits, and I was experiencing a shift beyond just the physical. It appeared to be quieting my mind, producing a level of clarity unknown to me before, and it healed parts of my heart that I never thought could heal through this method. It touched my soul.

CELLULAR SHIFT

Releasing Stressful Thoughts

Physical imbalances are often connected to emotions tied to mental states held captive inside of us. Mind-body-soul motivational author Louise Hay, known for her affirmations, spoke to this issue when she connected our perceptions and emotions to our physical state. With negative thoughts, we prevent a free flow of energy. This leads to disease, and disconnect in our body and mind.

During panchakarma, the release on the seventh night of the protocol purges the body *and the brain* of toxins, reducing inflammation. All five senses are heightened as the debris is flushed away. From the ayurvedic perspective, it is through our senses that we view the world, bringing data to the mind. Through the senses, we either cleanse or poison the mind. With PK, the cleanse supports the mind.

Each one of us faces challenges that manifest on the physical level but often are held under lock and key on an emotional level. My particular challenges at this time of my life were from perimenopause—discomfort from painful menstrual cramps, excess bleeding during my periods, facial breakouts like I was a teenager.

But discomfort soon escalated to life-threatening illness: a possible tumor on my ovaries. I got the message via voicemail. CA-125 blood work showed elevated levels of a cancer antigen. There it was—the cold, hard news, on a recording on my phone. I might have ovarian cancer. It was frustrating to receive medical information like this in such as thoughtless manner. I felt overwhelmed, in shock about what this might mean for my life. For a while, I carried a lot of fear and struggled to sleep at night. No one in my family ever had this kind of cancer. One of my first thoughts was of Gilda Radner, the Saturday Night Live comedian. Her ovarian cancer was discovered quite late, and she died. Research confirmed this was often the case. Ovarian cancer has few symptoms.

For a while, until I could get another test, I stayed in prayer and continued my yoga/meditation practice, which helped immensely. I shared this scary information with close friends, and doing this diffused the fear. Soon I was able to step back into a place of action as to what I needed to do next. At that point, I had an ultrasound, which showed I did not, in fact, have ovarian cancer. I was out of the woods, but not completely: I was told I need to be monitored for a period of time.

TENDER LOVING CARE

The Gift of Time

Give time to yourself throughout the day. Be aware. Be still for short periods of time. This increases the effectiveness of nurturing yourself. Lasting benefits are seeded in the daily rituals you offer to the body and mind. How do you nurture yourself daily?

It became quite clear that an integrative-medicine approach would be my path. In the last few years leading up to this time, I had been profoundly affected by the many losses in my personal and professional life. I have lost seven women psychiatrist friends, including two women in my private practice, to cancer in my twenty years in Albuquerque. Each one died of a different type of cancer, but the pattern did spur me to consider what it was about the work of women psychiatrists and the impact on their bodies, minds, and souls that has this effect. With each loss, I had to face my own mortality as a woman in a stressful field, one that has dramatically changed since I entered the practice. This signaled me to look more closely at my approach to my work. What stressors contributed to my perimenopausal symptoms and to the elevated blood test? Despite making numerous changes in how I approached my medical practice, I still wondered—were there issues that I still needed to address?

After confronting my own mortality, my desire for healing intensified. I had been evolving toward an ayurvedic lifestyle, but now I truly wanted to experience the depth and magic of Ayurveda. That brought me to Shalmali Joshi, who has training in gynecological Ayurveda, and is the wife of Sunil. I came to her before having one of the PKs. We decided to allow the herbs (which were recommended for treatment) support me for a month, then to have the PK.

After this particular panchakarma, I became more acutely aware of how it began the huge shift my body, emotions, mind, and spirit needed in order to ease into menopause with fewer symptoms. I noticed that I was weathering the day-to-day emotional shifts so much better. The more I changed my diet and incorporated other lifestyle changes, the more I experienced a sense of peace and well-being. I felt more balanced. My body felt more balanced, as did my mind and emotions. When the CA-125 test was repeated on two occasions, I got a clean bill of health.

But then I noticed something else: Harmony. The PK, along with the lifestyle changes, created a harmony for me that I wanted to keep. So my question became how to maintain this. I understood it would require my undivided attention, and so, I would go to India.

Introduction

Perhaps, like me, you have tried many things. Perhaps you have made many tweaks in your diet, exercise regimen, and daily habits over the years, seeking the optimum combination. Or perhaps you have tried on this spiritual teaching or that therapeutic technique in the hope of releasing old patterns and healing wounds in a way that creates lasting change. Each may have benefitted you by changing parts of yourself. And yet...

You still seek the profound transformative experience.

What if this method was faster and more sustainable than ten years of therapy? What if you could change your habits to healthier ones and heal parts of your wounded self that remain vulnerable? Imagine these changes occurring without great effort on your part during an eight-day process.

And, what if it were loving, kind, compassionate?

What Is Panchakarma, Exactly?

Panchakarma is an extremely **supportive physical cleanse** that is excellent for those with chronic disease. As previously mentioned, it can be described as as detoxification treatment taking place over seven days with the eighth day deemed a day of rest, involving massage, herbal therapy, and other procedures. Few of us these days do not have a health challenge of some kind. Yet, there is an experience that is possible for those who do not have significant physical challenges. *Rejuvenation* is possible, in the deepest way that we currently know of on this planet. The roots of panchakarma were developed in an effort to deepen the spiritual experiences of those who were on a devoted path to connect with the Divine.

————

Rejuvenation is what our planet needs. Panchakarma is a tool that has been hidden but needs to be revealed during these turbulent times.

————

The cleanse process, which includes the healing food provided during this time, allows for gradual **release of toxins** that have accumulated in the body and brain. Before we begin on the journey to India, before you come along with me, take this Toxin Quiz so you can be clearer on what kind of toxins are harming you.

QUIZ

What Toxins Are Weighing You Down?

Toxins can be our dark thoughts, negative feelings, unhealthy foods, drugs, alcohol, or pollution from the environment. Anything we ingest or are exposed to that may be deemed harmful to the well-being of our body, brain, and spirit would be considered a toxin. Each day of the eight-day process of panchakarma unfolds deeper layers within the body and brain, gently releasing more layers of toxins.

This quiz directs you to assess your time allocation, your choices about food and alcohol or drugs, along with predominant qualities of your thoughts and feelings. It asks you to estimate the percentage of your time and attention being exposed to toxins.

Think about the thoughts that you have each day about yourself, the people around you, and the news in your world.

TOXIN ASSESSMENT	YOUR ANSWER
About what percentage of these thoughts are negative?	
On any given day, what percentage of your feelings are negative, coloring your life in a dark way?	

TOXIN ASSESSMENT	YOUR ANSWER
In any given day, what percentage of your food is processed, deep fried, or out of a box?	
Do you drink alcohol? Do you use recreational drugs? About how many drinks per day? Do you tell yourself that you need to do this to numb out the negativity of your day?	
About what percentage of your day do you spend time on electronics?	

TOXIN ASSESSMENT	YOUR ANSWER
Does your city have poor air quality?	
About how many hours a day do you spend reading, listening to, or watching news? Is it often on in the background?	
About how many hours a day do you spend with family in a positive, loving manner, without electronics being a part of the time together? Include an assessment of your typical dinnertime.	

TOXIN ASSESSMENT	YOUR ANSWER
What would be one small change you could make to reduce the daily toxin load?	

A GUIDE TO DEFINITIONS

Before we discuss toxins further, let's get a few definitions out of the way:

Ayurveda

Ayurveda is a 5,000-year-old healing and medicinal system, the most complete and complex in terms of achieving true health and well-being available to us at this time on this planet. The central tenet of Ayurveda is tuning into the person as a true individual defined by a constitution or functional intelligence (dosha) that addresses us at the spiritual (soul/ *atma*), mental (mind/*manas*), emotional (the senses/*indriyas*), and physical (body/*sharira*) level. This constitutional/functional intelligence is referred to as the doshas; *vata, pitta,* and *kapha.* The doshas can be assessed by the pulse, by screening questions, and by physical exam.

Ayurveda is based on one of the ancient yogic philosophies called Samkhya yoga. Samkhya yoga is also one of the paths of yoga described in the yogic text the Bhagavad Gita, where it is explained as the path of correctly discerning the principles, or tattva, of existence.

As a philosophical tradition therefore, Samkhya, which means "number" or "to count," is concerned with the proper classification of elements of *prakriti* (nature) and *purusha* (spirit). The goal of Samkhya yoga is for practitioners to realize the difference between the spirit, purusha, and matter, prakriti.

Dosha

Dosha is a Sanskrit word used to describe three dynamic metabolic states representing the five elements (space/ether, air, fire, water, earth) in the body. Foundationally, the element of space cannot be changed, and earth is difficult to change, yet air (wind), fire, and water are dynamic, as we see on the earth where we live. The dance of these three elements expressed through the doshas is unique to each person, influenced by genetics, lifestyle, and even our thoughts. Vata is a combination of air and ether, and pitta is a combination of fire with some earth and water, kapha is a combination of earth and water.

Dhatus

When we discuss the doshas, it is only natural to discuss the *dhatus*. *Dhatu* is hard to define in English. It can refer to tissues in the body but it also refers to the fluids present as well. And each technique of panchakarma impacts all the tissues and fluids in the body.

Gunas

Ayurveda's theory of the creation of the universe is through the Yogic Samkhya. The universe that we live in is influenced by the *gunas*, three phases of activity in creation known as Sattva, Rajas, and Tamas . These gunas are also qualities of the mind. All of life is engaged in this dance between the three gunas.

In the mind, the qualities face unique challenges in how they are expressed.

The creative mode is *sattva,* bringing life into manifestation. In the world, it represents what is made by our Creator and what we see around us. Think of spring and all that it brings forth in this creative phase. In the mind, it is represented by the capacity for equanimity, balance. This is the natural state of the soul. It is via meditation, yoga, and a balanced lifestyle assisted by PK that this state can be experienced and maintained.

The next phase is referred to as *rajas,* which builds and maintains what has just been created. In the world it represents the building and maintenance phase, what is made by our Creator, and what we see around us. Think of summer and how all that was created in spring is being maintained. In the mind, it represents the activity of our thoughts.

When *rajas* is complete, then *tamas* destroys, thus bringing the cycle to an end. This would be the destruction or ending of the action. Think of fall, with all coming to an end and winter being the inertia before the cycle starts all over. In the mind, it is the inertia that can set in when there is a lack of movement.

It is important to remember these phases, as they are universal and all-persuasive. Yet the dance exists primarily between tamas and rajas in our day-to-day lives. This is where our daily choices impact our ability to return to our natural sattvic state of being.

Guna/activity is present in all aspects of our lives.

The universality of the gunas comes into play with our choices. Certain activities, foods, and people fall into each of these categories and impact our ability to maintain balance. One example we all can relate to would be when we are experiencing the affection of our loved ones as we share a meal that is balanced and supportive for all at the table. The action between the family members with love present is sattvic. The love that is poured into the food that is prepared has both the rajas and sattvic qualities. The food that is consumed begins to nurture the body and mind yet there are tamasic by-products from the food that need to be eliminated.

Toxins and Chakras

There is a chakra connection that I find amazing and can serve as a guide in the healing process for you. My theory is that as long as the body is full of the *ama* (toxins) that we continually add into our body, its filters are increasingly unavailable. Think about your windows that are dirty through the winter, and then in the spring they are cleaned. Every time, I notice how much more I am seeing and how much light comes in now that the "windows" of my cells are clean. Truth, as my soul sees it, comes forth with little effort.

PK is a form of window cleaning that impacts our chakras. Once we are physically cleansed of the toxins to at least a minimum threshold, we can connect to the chakras more easily. And this would start with the foundational first chakra known as the *muladhara*. This is the most important chakra, as truly one needs to be grounded in this life, because it is from this place of groundedness that decisions are made for the support of you and those around you.

And once the first chakra is sufficiently cleansed, each subsequent cleanse can assist you with each sequential chakra. More than one chakra may be cleansed each time, as there are variables that probably impact that possibility.

There is something else that happens in this process which is quite interesting. The cleanse allows the body to return to a level of equilibrium, homeostasis, with the innate intelligence resuming control. When this happens, all the layers of the body are nourished, with the doshic balance (combination of three main bodily substances) aiding in the flow of nutrients.

There is harmony and coordination present in the four areas of our life: soul, senses, mind, and body. Health and happiness are possible.

When this shift happens, the senses, our mind, and our soul are able to be nourished as well. And the biochemical substance responsible for this process is referred to as Ojas. It is responsible for nourishing these nonphysical parts of ourselves. This process allows us to connect with a part of ourselves that can connect with the Divine. This is known as Atman or Universal Consciousness.

Stress, as we know, is expressed in our bodies and brains in ways that we are all too familiar with. In Ayurveda, this imbalance is known as a *vata* imbalance. The interventions to support the reduction of the symptoms and return to balance are ones best done daily.

DEFINITION

Vata Dosha Imbalances

When *vata dosha* is out of balance, we experience physical, behavioral, and mental problems, such as:

PHYSICAL

Constipation, dry skin, intestinal gas, muscle spasms, intolerance to cold and wind, irritable bowels

BEHAVIORAL

Restlessness, low appetite, insomnia, inability to relax

MENTAL

Worry, anxiety, short attention span, impatience, depression, an overactive mind

What makes panchakarma unique is that through it the very patterns that you have had in your life may be changed. Think of a habit that would be best released. It may very well be possible with panchakarma. A small example that I experienced soon after the first cleanse is that I lost the desire to have coffee daily. I find that it is too bitter now for me to consume. I still have coffee on occasion, and can enjoy it in the context of sharing with another person, but I no longer *need* it upon awakening.

Each time you experience a cleanse, the body and brain respond more quickly. The starting point does not go back to where it was when you had the first cleanse. The starting line has moved in your favor. Allow me to clarify this point: When you are first exposed to the cleanse, only a basic level of penetration or depth is possible. When you repeat this cleanse yearly, your body responds to the treatments more readily—for a number of reasons. This is most often because you changed your lifestyle, as well as because a certain number of toxins flushed out previously are now gone.

HOW IT WORKS

The Reset Point

With each subsequent cleanse, the body is able to respond more deeply to the effect produced. Each panchakarma is an opportunity for the body and brain to create a reset point. This is a way for us to generate new reset points in the midst of our hectic lives.

A study about the effects of PK published in *Scientific Reports* in February 2016 indicated that several metabolic markers associated with cardiovascular disease, elevated cholesterol, and inflammation are significantly reduced by the eight-day cleanse.

Up to a week or two before I do PK, I feel a shift in my body. My body knows it is in for a treat. Each panchakarma is an opportunity for the body and brain to create a reset point—a way to start afresh. Exceptions to this might include, for example, a person who chooses to not make the lifestyle changes to the diet, sleep, and stress patterns that helped to create the negative conditions in the first place. And yet, with each subsequent cleanse, people find it easier to consider the necessary changes.

———

Yes, it does become easier to be your authentic self. Greater clarity, creativity, emotional stability, calm, peace...all are possible. Who would not want this?

———

This cleanse will also enhance any spiritual practice or focus that you may have. The physical cleanse is most important as it allows for the release of emotional toxins as well as physical toxins. As you become clearer/less toxic in the physical and emotional body, the mental chatter settles down. Then access to a spiritual connection/practice in a grounded way is possible. It has been said that Buddha did not start to meditate until he had a solid hatha yoga practice, a startling fact I found most enlightening. Our bodies are our vehicles to experience this world. Being grounded in your body allows for you to have a safer experience as you enter different realms of spiritual travel or consciousness with your meditation over time. Through our senses, we have ways to interact with the world as the mind navigates its way.

The ungroundedness I see among those exploring spiritual traditions is unsettling. "Ungroundedness" is a term that I use to describe individuals disconnected from their bodies who often are seeking ways to avoid dealing with this most amazing vehicle. Many people desire to reach a spiritual connection but in the practices of their traditions, little is done to support their grounding as they reach for the Divine. Moving past our senses without awareness of the dangers of the spiritual journey leads to mental health issues. Ungroundedness can result in unsettled and difficult emotional and mental challenges. Spiritual practices can allow you to reach new heights. I have been asked to consult in various settings when a person has become ungrounded and mental/emotionally unstable in the setting. Few tools were offered to the groups to keep them more present and grounded. Often, they were asked to leave the program and seek more allopathic support. Yet, I see little is done assisting to tether the person in their body, this precious vehicle we have been loaned to experience on this planet. Not so with panchakarma.

WHY IT WORKS

Being Grounded

PK cleanses toxins at all levels of your being. I have noticed this to be true in my further internal exploration through my spiritual practice. Now, when I reach for the Divine, I come from a place of greater purity with less ego involved. The ego wants what it wants, when it wants it, regardless if it is good for you or not. It creates confusion for us.

As toxins are released, it's possible to reconnect to the senses and to your intuition. This refines your "knowingness" so that you can make the choice that's best for your body and brain out of the daily options available to you. For me, this has had a grounding effect on my whole being. As I have become more grounded or present in my body, reaching for the Divine increasingly comes from a place where I am more present and connected.

Bouncing Back

Life gives us its share of bruises and bumps. As we age, bouncing back from these bruises and bumps can be more difficult. Depending on our genetics and lifestyle, these factors further confound our ability to return to a *baseline of balance and health*. Here is an intervention that is an investment of a different kind—one that can return you to a level of health not thought possible by most conventional standards of treatment. If you knew there was an option available that would not just maintain your health but actually having a *rejuvenating effect* as well...why not do it?

HOW IT WORKS

Rejuvenation

PK assists us in regaining health as we age (who is not aging?), first by reducing the toxin load. To feel rejuvenated is to feel younger and have more vigor. That has been my experience. PK has enhanced my quality of life throughout the years. Lifestyle changes further amplify the changes that come with the cleanse. One study, conducted at Kripalu and published in *Scientific World Journal* in the mid-2000s, measured the effects of holistic health interventions in Ayurveda and panchakarma and found that lifestyle changes came about more easily after PK.

At one level, PK serves to induce a cleanse at the most profound depth in order to move towards a stage of spiritual opening, and yet it also takes care of the health issues that each of us can develop due to our particular lifestyle and genetics. Our lifestyle further supports the changes that manifest in PK.

If less suffering is possible in this lifetime, who would not seek out panchakarma to bring about this possibility?

Who Am I Now?

The changes that have manifested for me have been multilevel and multidimensional. I now have an increased capacity to instill lifestyle changes in my diet/food choices and incorporate a yoga practice into my daily routine. My meditation is deeper, and I have a greater ability to sit in meditation daily. I have a sense of presence and of being present that only increases with each subsequent PK. This development has also included an increased clarity and focus on what it truly is that I am interested in pursuing in this lifetime. I have also experienced a greater level of health and well-being that has given me more energy in my day-to-day life. I am able to be present with that which is in front of me more calmly, despite what may be confronting me. Being centered and acting from that place of core strength has become easier for me.

That said, I am also more aware of what I can no longer tolerate in my environment. There are strong moments of rejection that come from within my being and which can be daunting for myself and those around me, as I have been typically more of a peacekeeper, not one to stir up the waters with conflict. Yet I am no longer quiet when people violate my boundaries. Traversing these new waters has required me to be more aware of my different emotional states when my boundaries are crossed, and to tread more lightly in my reactions to these situations when they arise.

Calm and focused is my more common demeanor now.

Changing Patterns

We all have patterns of behavior that we either inherited or developed over a lifetime. These patterns become expressed in our being through our body and brain. Our thoughts, emotions, and physical movement are a reflection of these patterns. They are present even at the cellular level. In Ayurveda, they are called *samskaras*.

Scientists are becoming more aware of the role our lifestyle has on our genetic expression in our daily lives. There was a time when we thought that our genetic makeup was unchanging from when we were born. This is no longer the case. We have increased knowledge we can no longer ignore. It matters what we eat and how we choose to live our lives, the level of stress we have daily, and this impacts our genetic expression.

HOW IT WORKS

Chronic Disease

With chronic diseases such as rheumatoid arthritis, lung conditions, diabetes, and Parkinson's, studies increasingly show that chronic diseases are very much related to the foods we eat and the lifestyles we lead.

PK jump-starts healthier lifestyle choices by inducing truly deep cleansing involving all the cells of our body. Medical conditions whose physical expressions in the body have been reduced after PK include arthritis (*Journal of Ayurveda and Integrative Medicine*, 2017), lung conditions (*Ayu*, 2010), diabetes (*Ayu*, 2013), Parkinson's (*Ayu*, 2010) and most inflammatory conditions.

Yet, PK can assist us in our return to wholeness and to the essence of our being, our soul. What a gift this is! What an opportunity during these most challenging times!

My personal challenges are not that uncommon for the average person. We all have health issues as we age. It is part of the human condition. I hope you are already realizing you can consider holistic healing options instead of surgery and/ or medications that often do not treat the original problem but may provide symptomatic relief.

What I discovered on this journey was not just a deep healing of the tissues in my ovaries and my endometrium, but a healing that went beyond.

Eight Days to Soul Freedom

HOW IT WORKS

Eight Days, Customized for You

All panchakarma journeys begin with an eight-day process that has a rhythm and pattern that is customized specifically for the individual. The plan is tailored to the physical, emotional, mental, and at times, spiritual needs of the person. The ayurvedic practitioner determines the plan after assessing you.

Each day builds on itself, culminating with the cleanse happening on the evening of the seventh day. On the eighth day, the clinician makes a concluding assessment and determines what herbs you need afterward.

As this journey is specific to me, there are specific procedures I have not experienced personally as my health is such that they are not necessary. These include *vamana* and *raktamokshana* procedures. Vamana is a prescribed form of vomiting that is medically supervised to help eliminate excess *kapha* in the body. It is a way of releasing that specific form of *ama,* or toxins, from the body. *Raktamokshana* is a medically supervised therapeutic way of drawing blood from the body.

Each day of the journey exposes you to different types of bodywork that aid in preparing your body and brain for that last day. Some of these interventions can be done separately from the eight-day process. One such process would be the *shirodhara*. This is incredibly soothing to the nervous system. If you are a bit edgy and feeling stressed, this healing process, wherein warmed, herbal-infused oil is poured onto the forehead for a period of time, is quite soothing for jangled nerves. Simply having this done once a week may improve your capacity to balance the challenges of your daily life after PK.

HEALING OIL

Shirodhara

Shirodhara is the pouring of warmed, herbal-infused oil onto the forehead. It is particularly effective for treating the vata disturbances that can happen to all of us. This fifteen- to twenty-minute procedure is very calming to the nervous system. The effects can last for a few days. An ayurvedic practitioner can administer this in your community.

AYURVEDIC RITUALS

The Run-Up

Before you embark on an eight-day panchakarma cleanse, it is good to prepare. Daily habits can both prepare you on your journey to PK and further the impact it will have on you after. One of these habits is a daily oleation of your body with coconut and sesame oil, depending on your constitution. Most people can tolerate this combination easily. Just developing this one habit can be exceptionally gratifying and soothing before choosing to do PK. Many of the body treatments mentioned are offered in spas across the United States as stand-alone interventions or in combination with other treatments. For example, a shirodhara is often given after the body massage that I describe.

When you seek services from ayurvedic practitioners in various settings such as a spa, you'll find that many of the procedures described are often recommended but not a necessary part of the PK regimen. Many spas in the United States and in India offer variations. Certain protocols are best performed by an ayurvedic bodyworker/technician. Ask about the training of the person who works on you.

Traveling to India is no small task, but it can be done. However, the majority of what I will describe can actually be done in the United States. Several places in the US provide ayurvedic interventions like the ones described in these pages. Internationally, there are places in Europe and South Africa as well where similar services are provided. Again, it would be wise to ask about the practitioner's formal training, which can consist of a six-week practicum (at a minimum) all the way up to training from one to four years at ayurvedic schools in the United States.

•••

Three basic concepts underscore the approach, so elemental that some may feel fooled by the simplicity of the recipe:

FOOD IS MEDICINE. "Food" is not confined to the food we ingest. It is any input into our body and mind that has an impact on us. An example of how this translates into our daily life would be any sensory input: what we listen to day in and day out, who we are exposed to daily, where we are throughout the day.

DISEASE CAN BE PREVENTED WITH OUR DAILY LIFESTYLE HABITS. This particular issue makes headlines daily, informing our current diet and lifestyle. And it's alarming that even as western society becomes more informed, indigenous cultures that have adopted western food choices suffer. Data indicates that between 1995 and 2010, the rate of diabetes, hypertension, and obesity in certain segments of the Native American population rose to levels comparable to those seen in the rest of the West, at the same time as their lifestyle was changing from a more traditional to a more contemporary model . Throughout this book, we will explore lifestyle recommendations as I share my experience with PK. The week spent doing the cleanse is but a microcosm of how you can live each day as you return to your life.

LIFESTYLE PRESCRIPTIONS ARE SPECIFIC TO YOUR DOSHA. Lifestyle prescriptions from an ayurvedic perspective take into account that each of us is a unique individual with a specific constitution that changes for a number of reasons. The prescriptions end up being a route into the body and mind to create balance and harmony.

An example of this prescriptive change would be as follows: I have issues with phlegm/mucus production; the prescription is to remove milk/dairy products from my diet, use the neti pot and nasya oil to remove the mucous and lubricate the nasal passages.

The holistic perspective of Ayurveda is all-encompassing. Ayurveda takes into account the internal aspects of your ingestion and your inputs, of how food impacts your being or essence down to the molecular level, including the seventh day after your food has long ago been digested. Ayurveda sees the connection between the internal aspects and the gross, external aspects, such as in the belief that your facial features convey information about what dosha you are. Each piece of information helps with the puzzle that you present to the ayurvedic clinician.

DEFINITION

Prakruti and Vikruti

The doshas describe mental, emotional, and physical aspects as expressed uniquely by every individual. At birth, there is a constitutional expression that occurs, known as *prakruti*. Over time, we develop an additional constitutional expression through lifestyle, diet, and other factors that move us from that initial stage. This is *vikruti*. That shift is due to imbalances in the doshas, and that's what creates what we see as disease in the body. Any excess or deficiency in one or more of the doshas creates disease. With PK, you are able to return to being closer to the *prakruti*. Why is this important to attempt? We are most balanced in this lifetime when we are closer to our *prakruti*, and the dharma of our life being is more likely to be expressed. That makes us healthier and more whole, and thus closer to the Divine essence of our being.

The Three Doshas

As previously mentioned, the three doshas are vata, pitta, and kapha. Each has specific qualities for physical, emotional, and mental characteristics. We all have elements of each but more of one than the others. It is extremely rare for a person to just have one dosha. I have mostly kapha and pitta for my prakruti, but my vikruti is a dance between too much pitta and a need to calm the vata. Most recently, I am more able to express the kapha qualities that I carry. Slowly but surely, I am making my way back to my prakruti!

The doshas are in constant motion in relation to one another in the body. Maintaining a balance between them is truly a challenge for any of us. This is where Ayurveda assists us greatly. And PK further supports us. In conversation with Joshi, my understanding of the process is that a still point is created for the body and the brain at the end of the cleanse, "a pause" that allows the body to shift toward its healthiest baseline at that point. The doshas are as quiet as possible for a brief period, then the dance starts all over again.

There are many sites online where you are able to do a self-assessment. It is a useful tool to have in order to develop a better understanding of what imbalances you have and what dosha(s) you have. It is basic information, and not diagnostic, but it can help you lean toward interventions that can help reduce or calm certain characteristics that may be out of balance for you.

The Journey Begins

When I returned from the Esalen retreat, I was ready to make a plan. The pull was irresistible, and I knew there was no turning back. I was absolutely certain that I would create time and space for my being. I was ready to explore what I needed to do to let the next phase of my life unfold. It was exciting. I knew I was on the path of greater expression for my life. I just didn't know where it might lead. I didn't immediately know the path, but I did know that the combination of yoga, meditation, supportive lifestyle, and PK was magic. So, I just allowed the magic to happen and waited for the processes to reveal yet another layer of my being.

In November 2013, I discussed with Sunil Joshi the possibility of having my next PK in India. I had gone to India two years earlier for PK. He graciously invited me to come to Nagpur again. We often would speak about the depth and magic of panchakarma during my appointments with him over the years. Each time, my enthusiasm grew. Now it was time to go.

In 2014, I attended a Haiku poem workshop. Here I learned to love writing Haiku. Each chapter begins with a Haiku that overall reflected my experience.

Chapter One

The Power to Heal

**HEALING STRENGTH UNLEASHED
WITH ULTIMATE GANESHA
PANCHAKARMA PRIMED**

PASSAGE TO INDIA

Ganesha

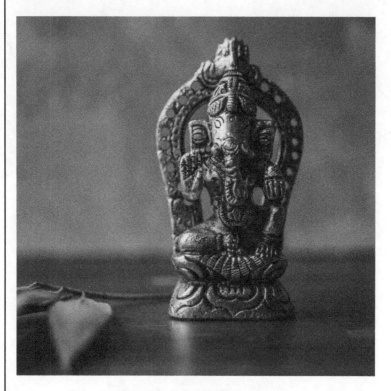

Ganesha, the Lord of Beginnings

Ganesha is the elephant-headed Hindu god known as the Lord of
Beginnings, sometimes as the Lord of Good Fortune. He is known as
the Remover of Obstacles of material and spiritual kinds. He may be
invoked each day to aid the release of obstacles, but we need to be
willing to surrender. He is also seated in our first chakra, helping to
ground us on this journey called life.

DAY ONE

Nagpur, India

Nagpur itself is in the center of India. During British colonial rule, it was the British government headquarters for all of India. The Vinayak Panchakarma Chikitsalaya clinic is near a wooded area along a street with well-maintained, large colonial buildings. Near the clinic, it is easy to walk the neighborhood and experience the street life of India, including the sacred cows that wander among the local people going about their day's business. Down the street is a laundry dobie, complete with a person who irons clothes right there on the street. At a Krishna temple nearby, a family tends the temple. The pace of life here is part of the healing rhythm. Yet I know the cocoon of the clinic awaits me.

I arrive at the clinic on a Sunday morning via a flight from Mumbai, after traveling nearly twenty-eight hours from the United States. I am fatigued but feel ready to start the process. I arrive in time for breakfast, and I am warmly greeted by several familiar faces, including Sunil's brother, Mukul, and the front-office staff. They show me to my room and then I come out for breakfast.

Neetu, who has been the cook for four years, is busy preparing the food. She greets me with a smile that has a glinting golden tooth. Her long, hennaed hair is pulled back. Her sari is a colorful green with vivid patterns of flowers. We navigate our communication with my limited Hindi and her growing knowledge of English. Gesticulations with our hands work as well.

Neetu serves me a savory farina accented with cilantro. She offers me a second portion but I decline. Ginger tea is hot and ready in the large container on the counter. Condiments are limited to salt and pepper, slightly spicy chutney, and freshly ground sesame seed with salt, cumin, and turmeric.

As I finish my breakfast, Neetu begins the preparation of lunch, which consists of rice and cooked vegetables with mild savory spices, dal (a soup made with lentils), and chapati (an unleavened flatbread). Each are placed in one-cup-sized, round stainless-steel containers with lids. They stack on top of each other and then are placed in the plastic thermos with the help of a stainless steel stacker. This whole set is referred to as a *tiffin*. The tiffin helps to keep the food warm and allows Neetu to do other things for that part of the day.

Given our varied schedules, lunch can be anytime from noon to 2 p.m. Once prepared, the tiffins are placed on the counter with our names. Due to many dietary restrictions, including specific diabetic or food-sensitive diets, an individual meal plan is needed for each person. Due to the increase in gluten sensitivity, teff (a wheat-free, gluten-free alternative grain, originally from Ethiopia) is offered for the chapatis (yeast-free bread) when needed.

I remind myself of what lies ahead.

CELLULAR SHIFT

The Two-for-One Cleanse

PK is a physical cleanse that detoxifies and rejuvenates the brain and body. It is a total cleanse that supports the body and brain and allows for a level of rejuvenation that has an anti-aging effect on the body. This process reduces ama (toxic waste that builds up in the body and brain due to poor diet, aging and stress). PK helps the body to recapture its ability to self-heal as it once did when we were younger.

Establishing a Routine

Each day is full, with body treatments starting early in the day, and for those inclined, an hour of yoga at 7 a.m. led by a staff member at the center.

It is so very important during the week to support the body and quiet the mind with breath work. The focus of the yoga at this clinic, and in general, is to aid in your digestion and to loosen up the joints...big and small.

Daily practice is started with an invocation to the guru (teacher) of your choice in addition to Krishna, as he is considered the father of yoga in this part of India. We share this in a seated position of our choice, but typically it is on our knees on the floor. This sets the tone of what we are asking for as we start the practice of yoga.

Instructors teach breathing exercises with meditation at the end of the class. They recommend that we do them two times daily.

YOGA SPOTLIGHT

Child's Pose

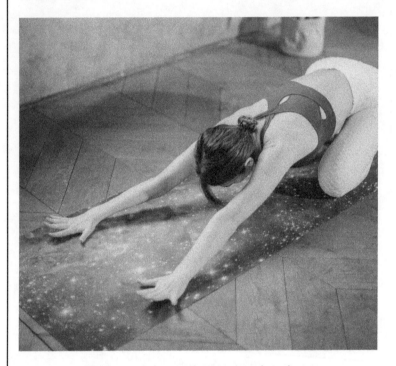

Child's pose helps you slow your breathing down.

This deceptively simple pose of kneeling down and placing your forehead on the ground (or as close as you can) sets the tone of surrender that will be a theme as the week unfolds. Having our head below our heart encourages deference to the healthy needs of the body. This posture is recommended when you need to slow breathing down in the practice or simply to rest. It aids in reducing external stimuli as well. It is easier to achieve a quiet mind and body.

We are provided with all our meals. They are cooked on site with an ayurvedic approach—translation: minimal to no spicing, minimal oil and use of ghee (clarified butter), no processed food, essentially vegan but maybe milk with tea (this was a slight change when I was there the last time...chai with ginger is now allowed in the morning only!), no coffee, and certainly no alcohol or smoking. The cook's demeanor is quite sweet and she is there twice daily to prepare our meals, which are, again, placed in tiffins. The tiffin keeps the food hot and separated, and includes rice, a cooked vegetable and dal, and of course, *rotis* (a wheat flatbread made fresh with no yeast). Sunil Joshi aids in making sure that dietary needs are addressed, including for diabetics. It is best to avoid rice during this time.

FOOD AS MEDICINE

Cilantro

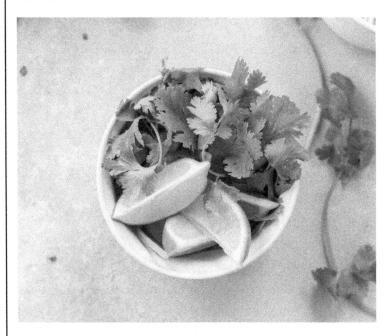

Cilantro releases heavy metals from the body.

Cilantro (*Coriandrum sativum*) is in the Apiaceae family, along with parsley, celery, and parsnips. The dried herb is referred to as coriander. As a fresh herb, it is used in Asian and Indian cuisine as a garnish. In its fresh form, rather than its dried form, it is one of the best herbs to aid in releasing heavy metals from the body. Cilantro eases stomach upset as well. It has anti-inflammatory, antiviral, and antibacterial effects on the body.

The ayurvedic approach to food includes fresh, nicely spiced rice with cooked, lightly spiced vegetables. Cilantro is served as a garnish with each meal. Cilantro is one of the most supportive herbs gifted to us, as it aids in detox, especially of heavy metals. It also reduces gastric upset.

The ayurvedic approach to food is fresh with both dried and fresh herbs to enhance the healing qualities of the food.

We take herbs in tinctures and pill form to further prepare the body and brain for the process overall. Some support digestion and elimination as well, to improve quality of sleep. In addition, you are asked to take a certain amount of medicated ghee in the morning and at 4 p.m.—noting when your appetite returns after having taken it. This is gradually increased to an amount appropriate for you. This is only the beginning—the goal for the week is to introduce enough oil in and on your body to facilitate the final purge on the eighth day.

Some come for a month for the repeated process. It is always an eight-day process unless the person in question has a specific problem to be addressed. One Indian woman with amazing long white hair and colorful saris, age sixty-four, was there to seek help with her knees to avoid surgery. She is doing much better after the six months of treatments she received. With these regular treatments, she has experienced much less pain and is able to walk now. She has been going there for several months and stays for a number of days for the process. She said that the name of the process should be prema-panchakarma. Prema means "love." I could not have said it better.

HOW IT WORKS

Just for You: Personalized Medicine at Its Best

The bodywork for PK is general in some areas, but specific to your health needs in others. For example, I am given a certain protocol that will be modified each day. Another person with pre-diabetic issues is given limited rice and more vegetables. The steam box is not offered to the person who is suffering low blood pressure. A person sensitive to oil may have ghee applied during the massage.

I am given a daily intake form to fill out that addresses how I am feeling, how much medicated ghee I took, when my appetite returned, how many bowel movements I've had and when, and how I slept. Here I note issues and then the clinic director, Joshi, addresses them.

After breakfast, I arrive for morning body treatments. I slip under the sheet and take a deep breath as two massage therapists begin to work on me with heated oil and herbs.

Two massage therapists work on me with heated oil and herbs. The process starts to get the body ready to release toxins via the skin by sweating and via the gut with gentle cleansing or oil enemas. They gently steam my skin to further drive in the oil. Then a small amount of medicated oil is placed in each nostril which helps to cleanse and release whatever is in the nasal passages. Next, they place me in a steam box for three to four minutes. Given each person's individual constitution, specific remedies are given. For me, lower back issues can be present, so I was given a herbed-oil *basti* on the lower back. The enema is given at the end, and you are asked to hold it to the best of your ability for as long as you can.

All this can take about one to one and a half hours to complete. Some days, they saw up to eleven people a day. And yes, you are quite oiled up in the end! The good thing is that the clinic had the foresight to place solar panels on the roof for the water heater, thus there is always plenty of hot water.

To finish the day—usually by late afternoon—if so indicated for you, they give you a shirodhara, which is a warmed, herbed sesame oil that they gently sweep across your forehead. Yes...more oil again, but it's well worth it. The benefit of this intervention is that it calms the mind/brain down, and this is incredibly true. Sometimes, I fall asleep or go into a very quiet, calm space inside.

Before We Begin

Practitioners review your clinical history to see if you are still a candidate for PK. They take an ayurvedic pulse to determine the state of your constitution now relative to your birth constitution. They take an ayurvedic pulse just like any other pulse, but there are layers to the pulse allowing the practitioner to assess the doshas. This helps them to understand how much of an imbalance is present at this time.

Once they determine that you are clinically stable, they give you a prescription for specific herbs, which goes to the herb clinic on site. This includes tonics to start the rejuvenation, herbs to further aid digestion and elimination, as well as other treatments specific to your constitutional imbalance. One example is the *Dadim* herb tonic. It is made with pomegranate and aids reduction of acid in the stomach. It is most pleasant tasting!

A Plan

Sunil greets me with a big smile as I enter his office. "So glad you made it here from the US. It is quite a privilege to work with those who make the trek to India for the panchakarma! Here we have more herbal options for you, as many of the best herbs are delivered most effectively in tinctures."

My curiosity piqued, I asked, "What prevents you from offering them in the US?"

"Custom restrictions prevent liquids from entering the US in a timely manner!"

Sunil reviews the plan of action with me. I would have three liquid herbs after lunch and dinner, each having a different function: *Sup. Amlapitta*—to aid in pulling out excess heat/pitta; *Sup. Abhaya*—to aid in pulling toxins/ama out; and *Sup. Dadim*—which is made with pomegranate and aids in pulling acid from mucous membranes. I would also have three different tablets after lunch and dinner: *Livotone*—which supports the liver; *Pittashamak vati*–which draws out ama out in balanced manner; and *Tager*–which aids in calming vata dosha.

At bedtime, I was given *Avi* powder, which is dissolved in warm water and further pulls out excess pitta, as well as *Sup. Brahmi*, which supports the neurotransmitters/peptide production in the brain, *drishti* eye drops to reduce pitta, and medicated ghee (*tikrita*), which is taken in escalating doses throughout the week, two times a day (in the morning and at 4 p.m.). Once taken, it is important to note when appetite returns.

Daily personal oleation is also practiced to further calm down vata and releases more ama.

Seeking Calm

From this list of herbs, it's clear that Sunil sees a need to calm the vata and pitta part of my body and mind. He does not see any huge physical issues that I am dealing with at this time, but there are specific physical sites that the herbs are to address. This includes hip discomfort due to an imbalance in my hips from a previous Achilles tendon repair.

Sunil then takes my blood pressure and pulse. He listens to my lungs and heart with the stethoscope, then palpitates my abdomen. I have tenderness in one area of my abdomen, in the lower right quadrant. My blood pressure is the normal range. I am clinically stable enough to have the treatment, he announces.

CONTRAINDICATIONS

When Not to Do Panchakarma

A clinical assessment can include your emotional state. Through conversation the practitioner assesses if you are emotionally stable enough to begin the procedure. Sunil has shared with me that if you have evidence of mania (agitated, elevated mood states in bipolar disorder), this would be a contraindication to start the process.

Other conditions that would prevent you from starting PK include: your menstrual period (schedule the treatment when you are not going to be on your cycle); persistent elevated blood pressure; intestinal bleeding.

We discuss the goals for my PK this time. There is a spiritual/emotional component that will be the focus. "Judith," he says to me, "your treatment is to take you deeper into your heart, as we will open your heart chakra even more, in order to balance your inner planes of being and the external expression of them. I want you to be able to express your consciousness more fully."

———

Remember that with each cleanse, there is a
deeper access to your inner being that impacts
the spiritual and emotional parts of you.
Much release is possible if you surrender.

———

At this point, I am near tears as I hear Sunil's words. I have so many thoughts and feelings running through me. I am feeling overwhelmed and jet lagged from the long journey, yet I am also excited to hear what he is saying. It is so close to the mark of what I am seeking. My eyes begin to well up with tears—tears of joy and gratitude for being here in Nagpur. I feel that I am truly seen through the eyes of Dr. Joshi. He has some understanding of my intentions to deepen my connection with the Divine, to really be able to express my inner being with the world at large, to share the beauty that I experience when I connect with the Divine. It can be as simple as going on my favorite walk on the acequia, experiencing the beauty of the sunsets over the volcanoes, watching the dragonflies flit over the water, hearing the ring-necked pheasant in the distance and occasionally seeing it nearby the walking area. The sunlight as it dances over the water and on the side walls of the acequia in the morning. In it, I feel such magic in being present and being able to see, hear, smell, and touch life and all the elements of nature as it is.

After the consult, I emerge to see Pravin summoning me to come for the start of treatment. He is the lead ayurvedic technician. He has been trained by Sunil. His love of what he does is quite palpable.

"It is time for you to be on the table. You are next...did you miss us?" Pravin asks with a big, warm smile.

"Of course I did," I say as I give him a hug.

As I undress in one of the treatment rooms, I feel anticipation and excitement as to what the week will unfold for me. Placing my face into the cradle of the massage table and covering myself, I feel my body begin to relax more and more. I have noticed that my body is more quickly primed to the process each subsequent time. Ready and waiting as is my mind and soul.

Here I am again, but I feel different from the first time. I am more aware of the rhythm of the clinic. I see there is little change with the staff and notice how at ease I am with each person. I am able to surrender to the process of the cleanse as I know what is going to happen—and yet I also don't. I do know what procedures are to happen but I do not know how my mind, emotions, and body will respond. Each time is different. My needs change each time, my response does as well.

What is possible this time? I feel the need to talk but know it is not time. Keeping a level of quiet is important now. I am able to travel into my interior world as the external world recedes. Less sensory stimulation adds to the process of turning inward.

TENDER LOVING CARE

A Double Massage (Bahya Snehana)

Bahya snehana refers to the massaging of warm, herbed sesame oil into the body. The process starts with warmed oil placed in a certain sequence on the body, and then two individuals commence in following how the prana is thought to flow in the body. They match each other in the strokes and rotations of their hands. This continues throughout the time they are applying the oil.

This is both relaxing and intense because the rhythm and pattern aids in calming the vata state and releases tension in the body and mind. The pattern of movement is similar on both sides of the body and follows the pattern of how the doshas move on the surface areas of the body. For example, to aid in digestion, movement clockwise happens over the abdominal area in a gentle manner.

Oleation (Snehana)

There are several ways of applying oil to the body externally and internally. This includes the nose with *nasya* (herbed oil). Later, the process of basti, consisting of enema treatments and external placement of warm, herbal oils over focused areas of the body, will be discussed. The intention is to aid in pulling the ama into the digestive tract and to ease elimination of toxins as the week progresses.

One internal oil that is given is medicated herbal ghee (clarified butter), referred to as *tikrita ghee*. Depending on the state of your constitution, you start with one-fourth to one-half of a teaspoon of this specific ghee twice a day—in the morning upon awakening and then at 4 p.m. The dose is increased as you are able to tolerate it. You wait until your appetite returns (which is a sign that you have digested the ghee) to have a meal.

In addition to the herbs you are taking with meals or at bedtime, you are given herbed oil to be applied to your own skin at a separate time from the bodywork. After applying the herbed oil, you allow it to remain on for about five to ten minutes, which will deepen the beneficial aspects of the procedure as the oil is able to be absorbed into the body. You can take a shower or bath to remove the excess afterward. I typically use a paper towel to absorb the excess and have had fewer clogged drains as a result of this simple step. This daily application of oil is referred to as *personal abhyanga*. I, and many others, practice this oleation daily while in PK. What I have noticed is that my skin feels wonderful afterward. I am calmer and I notice that I am more present. It is quite nurturing to self-soothe with the massage, and I also find the process to be grounding.

Our skin is our largest sensory organ. It perceives our environment in many ways beyond just touch. I learned this in discussion with Dr. Joshi, and have noticed it more since, be it the temperature in the room or the sense of feeling safe in a space (or not). Who has not experienced their hair standing on end in the face of fear? Nurturing your skin with this oleation process is truly a gift to yourself.

DAILY AYURVEDIC RITUALS

Personal Abhyanga (Oleation of the Body)

Personal Abhyanga is an important daily habit to develop because it:

- Nurtures you as the warmed oil is applied to the body (remember that skin welcomes touch, including our own; our skin is the largest sensory organ that we have)
- Calms the nervous system
- Improves circulation
- Softens the skin
- Pulls out ama from the body
- Gives you and your body, when *done daily*, a gift that keeps giving all day long

Bodywork

The ancient protocol commences. The process starts on the back and then down the arms, then both legs. Then I rotate face-up, so the attendants can begin the process with my abdomen, then my chest, arms, and legs. This is very different than a typical massage because of the patterns they follow and because there are two people massaging you simultaneously. This type of massage is typically very relaxing, but some might find it invigorating as well.

The intention of the massage with the oil is to begin to pull the ama from the skin and into the digestive tract, as well as to saturate your skin with the oil. The skin is the largest organ of elimination. Much absorption of oil is possible during this week. The amount of oil absorbed is relative to each person but a certain amount is needed for effective release to happen on the eighth day.

That is in fact the goal. Typically, the ayurvedic practitioner conducts a little pinch test to determine if you have absorbed enough oil into your skin. I had no idea about the importance of this until the last day of the procedure. When Dr. Joshi pinched my skin after he viewed my tongue, I asked about the pinch and he explained.

HOW IT WORKS

Nadi Swedana

The next body treatment is *nadi swedana*, a hand steaming of your skin. The ayurvedic bodyworker uses a hose producing steam (not too hot) to follow the pattern of the external oleation and of your own *abhyanga*. The attendant applies steam to the back, then the front, which further drives the oil into the skin. Wet heat is very good for the joints of the body. The treatment can be given beyond PK to treat back pain as well as inflammation of the hips and knees.

Nasya is the process of applying warm, herbal oil into the nasal passages after a practitioner gently rolls a hot-water bottle over your face. The nose and sinuses are then massaged to further drive the oil inside the nasal passages.

DAILY AYURVEDIC RITUALS

Nasya

Personal *nasya* is a practice you should continue afterward because it helps to limit accumulation of pollen and other particles in the nasal passages and offers lubrication/moisture. This is a good, proactive move for those with allergies and chronic sinus issues. This practice is simple. Apply a few drops in each nostril as you tip your head back and massage the upper nose area. Keeping the head back or simply supine for a brief period of time assists in keeping the oil in the nasal passages. If you use a neti pot first to cleanse the passages with a warm saline solution, this removes the pollen and congestion in the nasal passages. This is a basic practice for nasal hygiene. This simple intervention aids in reducing sinus issues, including infections.

After the nasya treatment, I receive a facial and scalp massage, with even more oil. At this point, the bodywork is done for the day. A steam box nearby is like steam sauna, but this particular model allows for your head to be above and outside the box. The process is referred to as *baspa swedana*. Before I sit in the box, an attendant brings me a glass of water. Initially, I find being in the steam box to be relaxing, then as the heat builds, it can be more of an endurance test to stay in there beyond a few minutes. That appears to be the experience of most people. If you remain in the box for about five to six minutes maximum, you can generate a nice sweat to further release toxins in the body. Remember that the skin is our largest elimination organ.

HOW IT WORKS

Baspa Swedana

Baspa swedana is a form of steam sauna that further aids detoxification. Unique to this process is that your head is outside of the steam box. You are placed in the sauna for about six minutes.

A cautionary note: some medical conditions cannot tolerate this procedure. Those with heart disease and hypertension can find their heart rate increased as well as their blood pressure, in which case the *nadi swedana* will be sufficient.

Afterward, I take a quick shower to wash off any oil that did not come off in the steam box. I always feel very relaxed at this point and almost spent. This time, I notice my skin feels very soft and hydrated. I am glowing inside and out, which sends a thrill through me. The attendant gives me a warm herbal mixture with which to gargle. There is an astringent quality to the taste, but I note that this will further aid detox for me. It will draw out my ama.

Each intervention works in tandem with all the ways the body has to eliminate waste from it, and typically, it is done in a gentle, effective manner.

"Cooked" and Invigorated

For the most part, the morning body interventions are completed for this first day. Often, practitioners will choose to use one or two different basti (therapeutic herbed oil placed on skin or into the colon for specific reasons) but not always on the first day. Colon basti are the exception. More on basti later!

By this time, like many people on their first day, I am pretty "cooked." I feel tired but also invigorated. I know that resting is most important even though I feel energized. Each day will present its own challenges at all levels, so it is important for me to pace myself and not push too hard.

As the sun is setting, shadows deepen in my room. It becomes darker in the clinic as we get closer to 6 p.m. I feel the desire to reach out to those at home but realize that it is still early in the United States. I am a bit sad about not being able to text as easily as in the US. I decide to send emails to my family to let them know all is well and that I arrived safely. As it is Sunday, I do not have many emails to respond to as yet. I also am realizing the precariousness of internet access. It is only available in certain public areas of the clinic and can be difficult to connect to on the floor I'm staying on. Little did I know, this challenge would only increase.

I have finally been able to email my daughter, sharing with her that all is well. I hear all is well for her too. It feels good to connect with her, and I am finding the email sufficient for now. When timing the emails it is important to remember as there is an eleven-and-a-half-hour difference between here and the US. The schedules of those back home are in exact opposition to mine. This is less so for the Europeans here, as it is only about seven to nine hours difference for them.

As the evening turns to night, I share a cup of ginger tea after dinner with my friends. I share my internal journey of the last few months that led to the external journey to India. I am feeling a strong tug to shift directions in my career. I had been on a walk earlier in the day with the one East-Indian couple at the center when a conversation about this had begun Prakesh heard me and said, "Jump off the train!" As we spoke more about this concept, I heard him explain, "There is a time for each of us, if we are listening, to think about simply jumping off the train we have been on most of our lives. I did the same. Twice! Now it is your turn!"

DAILY MORNING RITUALS

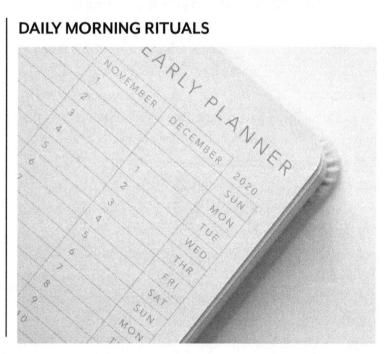

Note: A blank ritual journal is provided in the Appendix.

ROUTINES	Rise early enough to have time to incorporate the practices of self-love and tender loving care.
OIL	Practice oleation of the body with warmed, herbed oil before the morning cleansing ritual.
CLEANSES	Scrape tongue with tongue scraper.
FOOD AS MEDICINE	Prepare fresh-grated ginger tea. Choose breakfast foods that are best for your health status.
MOVEMENT	Engage in early morning exercises of ten to twenty minutes, a simple yoga routine, stretching, walking or running outdoors.
MEDITATION	Establish a meditation/contemplation practice. Sitting from five to twenty minutes in the morning aids in centering the mind to prepare for the day.

Chapter Two

•

Day of Transition

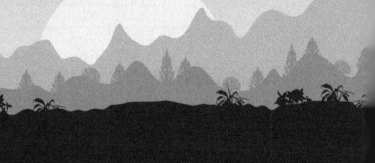

INTENSE BODYWORK
OLEATION, STEAMING, HERBS
INCLUDE ORIFICES
UP AT 2 A.M.
MIND ALERT, BODY DRAINED
MULLING, RELEASING

DAY TWO

I awaken with the morning dawn near 6 a.m. Despite having woken up at 2:30 a.m. for about an hour, I am feeling less fatigued. I begin the morning ablutions. The routine includes scraping my tongue to aid removal of the ama that is being released in the body. I then take a shower. After that, I meditate using a yogic breathing technique known as *pranayama*. Often practitioners prescribe alternate-nostril breathing in yoga practice and in ayurvedic lifestyle regimens because it balances the right and left brain. These breathing techniques help to engage the parasympathetic (calming) part of the nervous system. This is a tool that many people continue to use after PK so they can maintain the calm that the cleanse brings. Today, I chose to do alternate-nostril breathing.

DAILY AYURVEDIC RITUAL

TONGUE SCRAPING

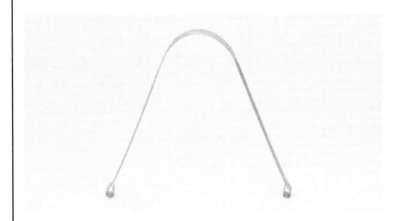

Tongue scraping removes *ama*.

Tongue scraping is an easy intervention done with a tongue scraper made out of stainless steel or copper. In my experience, the plastic tongue scrapers appear not to be thorough for cleaning the tongue. The tongue scraper removes *ama* that has built up on the tongue through the night. This is good for oral hygiene as well as overall health. It becomes part of the morning ritual.

I take herbs, then the medicated ghee. I start with one-fourth of a teaspoon. The ghee is liquid as it is warm enough here in India at this time to remain liquid.

Each morning at 7 a.m. the clinic offers yoga. On this day, I am the only student in the class. As I wait for the teacher, I notice that I feel rested, given my fatigue from travel and being up early after nine hours of sleep. In this moment, I feel ever grateful for having the opportunity to be back at the clinic. This time, I feel less overwhelmed in trying to keep up with the rhythm of a clinic in a foreign land.

The yoga teacher, Pritti, arrives. She is the wife of Mukul, who manages the clinic. She smiles a gentle smile when she sees my own. Given the formality of the moment, no hugs are exchanged. We begin the session with a simple mantra to recognize the guru who aids us in the practice of hatha yoga. At one point, we repeat the mantra for the honoring of the sun, *Suriya*, for all it offers to us day in and day out as we do six sun salutations.

YOGA SPOTLIGHT

Sun Salutations

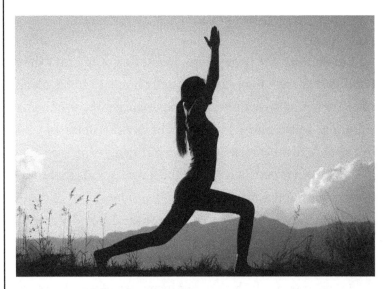

**The twelve movements of the sun salutations
lay the groundwork for lifelong vitality.**

These twelve movements/asanas are most supportive for your well-being. Daily practice of these specific asanas has a supportive and preventive impact on the body, keeping your spine supple and your joints moving. Learning this simple series may be sufficient for your overall health and vitality over a lifetime.

We do primarily standing poses with some twists, then eventually move to the floor. Pritti introduces more breathing practices for me to practice. Pritti offers cues as to when to bring them into my own personal practice. Eventually, three others join us, following the instructions to the best of their abilities. One elderly Indian couple make the modifications they need and remain for the hour.

—————

PK changes you from the inside
out. In eight days you are changed
in every layer of your body.

—————

As I move with the instruction, memories of my first time flood in. I cherish the sense of coming home to India, along with a sense of acceptance. I do experience a sense of being culturally overwhelmed in this land of intense contrasts, yet I feel an underlying connection to the spirituality expressed here in India, seen everywhere. From the flower stands that carry flowers for the temples, to the frequent placement of those temples in the communities. This allows the devoted person to simply stop by and ask for a prayer to be answered, or to simply offer respect to the deity represented there.

I sense how much I have grown in my own personal practice of yoga. In the intervening two years, I have developed a home practice in the United States. I have added yoga to my morning routine before I do my pranayama and meditation practice that I have had for more than twenty-four years. Yet Pritti shares mantras that are new to me. I welcome them.

Pritti has added movements specific for the joints. We stand at the top of our mats, place our fingers on top of our shoulders and rotate our arms. Later when we are doing the seated poses, we grab one foot and bring back the leg, keeping the calf of the leg perpendicular to the floor, then repeating this movement on the second side. We then rotate each hip several times in one direction then another. Each of these moves stimulate these large joints in the body to increase fluidity and mobility.

HOW IT WORKS

Kapalabhati Breathing

All the breathing techniques described in this book are best done in the presence of a teacher in order to receive the best instruction to support your state of health. Correct posture and an empty stomach are requirements.

Kapalabhati is known as the "breath of fire" as it invigorates your brain and body. It can support your sinus and respiratory health. It is a quick, strong breath in, with the inhalation happening passively. It can be done for a few seconds or for about a minute, even longer, if practiced regularly. This is another *pranayama/*breathing technique often incorporated into a daily meditation practice. It is very *good to stimulate the brain*. And as it does stimulate the brain, it is good to do this breathing earlier in the day. This is a way to wake up the brain... without coffee.

Always stop if you're feeling light-headed or faint. Only go as far as is comfortable for you.

At the end of the flow sequence, we start kapalabhati breathing. My sinuses felt great afterwards. When we finish, Pritti offers the option of meditation or *savasana*. Today I sit still and meditate. It feels right.

Breakfast follows soon after. This usually consists of a grain that is cooked in a savory manner. The garnish is cilantro, as it is for every meal.

My favorite breakfast happens to be the pancakes made of mung-bean flour and served with a mild coconut chutney. Neetu is all smiles when we praise her cooking. We all negotiate with her. "Neetu, is it possible to have a second serving of pancakes?" I ask.

"Yes, of course!" she replies with a grin. Ginger tea with fennel, cumin, and coriander, made fresh twice daily, is available throughout the day.

Often, up to ten people can be in the clinic receiving treatments at one time. The rhythm of mealtimes is determined by where you are on the schedule, which can change day to day. We share mealtimes in a scattered fashion for breakfast because of the tight schedule for the various modalities. Lunch is similar, as the treatments in the clinic may last until almost 1 p.m. Dinner is often shared with the group and can be quite a boisterous affair, as most of us have been pretty silent for the day. Conversation topics can range widely because of the international flavor of the group—patients from Switzerland, Germany, France, USA, and southern India. The group reflects the breadth of consultations that Sunil Joshi conducts in Europe and in the United States.

The time each person arrives for treatment periods reflects each person's unique healing process. This poses its own challenges, as it is rare that more than two or three people are in the same phase of treatment. When I arrive, five people had already been there for three weeks and were further into the process. I am entering my first week, an introspective week. I notice this mainly when I find my need for quiet pushed during the meals, though not always. The energy of the others is more outward, with lots of talking in very animated ways. I chose to eat upstairs on the rooftop during the day. I also consider eating in my room. Many are close to being finished in their treatment protocol, ready to go home when I am just starting.

One East-Indian couple start the same week I do. We quickly become each other's supporters. When we are all in a good space, we can easily become as silly and fun as the rest of the group, sharing stories of the changes that have come about with the power of PK.

THE DISH ON DOSHAS

A Kapha Dosha Issue

One East-Indian man in our group has a *kapha* imbalance. This dosha has the elements of earth and water, which impacts mucous production, that in his case, have led to chronic lung problems. He states that he came to the Nagpur clinic years ago and found the PK treatment very effective. He had returned because the condition had recurred.

I noted that had not returned until now, several years later. So the PK appeared to have had a lasting effect on him. He vowed that next time he would come back sooner, before his kapha dosha got out of balance.

The bodywork commences as the morning unfolds. It always starts with the external oleation. But today an extra procedure has been added due to the prescription that I have received. It is one of my favorites—*pinda swedana*. The ayurvedic technician takes a warmed-milk decoction and applies it with a soft rice bag onto your body similar to the way that the oil is applied. Only one person is applying the milk bath. This procedure is able to "tonify the muscles and improve circulation." These herbs aid in the flushing of the liver at a volume that most people tolerate. Afterward, I enter the steam box steam box for about three to four minutes. I shower and notice my skin is incredibly soft.

Basti

The next procedure is basti, either an internal or external placement of warm, herbed oil.

A basti is seen as nourishing not just the tissue it touches but also impacting the more subtle levels of the body in that area. The basti impact ama and other toxins present in the *dhatus*.

The power of the basti cannot be overestimated. Basti have the capacity to bolster the beneficial changes of panchakarma up to 50 percent compared to the other procedures defining PK as noted by Joshi.

After the shower, I move to a clean massage table to have the basti, and depending on where it is placed, this determines whether you are face up or face down. The ayurvedic technician places the basti on the external areas of the body that need special attention, based on the clinical assessment at the beginning of the week.

An example of a basti would be placing warm oil with herbs on the sacrum area. The ayurvedic technician first places down a ring of handmade dough, creating a circle over the sacrum. Securing the edges of the dough inside and outside, the technician pours oil in this circle of dough. This supports and nourishes areas that may have pain or other problems such as stiffness.

Many basti are possible, and it depends on your conditions noted at the initial consult. For me, because of lower back issues and tension in my neck area, they give me the one for the sacrum and one for the upper back and neck region. I find the second procedure on my neck can be quite a challenge because

I have to stay perfectly still so as not to have the oil start leaking or spill out of the dough vessel that is hand-created each time by the ayurvedic technician. Once, I did move and I could feel the oil running down my neck. I simply smiled and attempted to remain still for the rest of the treatment. It is really the only time when you are "in charge" of the way the process goes for the fifteen minutes you are face down. The heart basti is not as difficult because there is only one dough circle used, and I find I am not as inclined to want to move as when I have the two basti on my back.

These herbal and/or herbed-oil basti are seen as nourishing the tissues deeper than at the skin level. This is significant to note, as many of us have had colonics/enemas for health reasons. An enema or colonic, which is water-based only, can be depleting for the colon and body.

This process can be healing for the tissues of the body because of the absorption of medicated oils. Thus, basti done as part of the PK process aid in pulling toxins from the body as the oil goes through the entire length of colon, and beyond as the herbs and oil are absorbed by the body. In this way, *basti* impact all the *dhatus* and doshas and are an excellent way to calm the vata imbalance that a person can experience. The oil has a restorative aspect, providing nourishment to the tissues of the colon.

THE DISH ON DOSHAS

Vata Disorders

Disorders that have a vata component include arthritis, constipation, sciatica, lower back pain, and rheumatism. Basti can help certain neurological conditions as well. Basti can aid in reducing the discomfort associated with these conditions. There are conditions for which basti are not to be given, including diarrhea, colon cancer, and rectal bleeding.

Elimination

There are few places in our daily lives in which we can share about our elimination, or speak about private challenges that we might have with elimination. Here, with the gathering of people you have been sharing space with for the past several days, bowel movements can often be a topic of conversation as well as a source of laughter. This is mostly based around the challenge of the internal basti. The attendants introduce internal basti into the rectum at the end of the morning procedures. The day I receive a nourishing basti is a less challenging day. The time that follows is often one of the "free times" of the day. Many of us have a desire to walk at that time, but woe to the person who travels too far from the clinic. The releasing of the bowels has a timing all of its own...often quite unpredictable, it can be as soon as ten minutes or as long as an hour. With the nourishing oil-based basti, it is easier to leave the clinic, as it does not stimulate the bowel as much as the more stimulating cleansing basti. Many moments of humorous emotional release can result from these close calls, as everyone becomes more comfortable with the results of these various interventions.

TENDER LOVING CARE

Internal Basti

Internal basti are oil infused with certain herbs or a water-oil base with herbs. The herb-based basti are more nourishing and less depleting than the typical colonics given in the United States, which are water-based and use no herbs. The basti further aid in pulling ama (toxins) from the deeper tissues beyond the colon back into the colon. The colon is one of the body's primary detoxifiers.

In Ayurveda, the colon is also another area where the vata dosha resides, so it is important to consume enough moisture/liquid as well as healthy oils in our diet. This prevents dryness so there is less risk of constipation.

One couple from Switzerland come almost yearly for a month-long process because the male partner had developed early diabetes. Now Peter comes more for the maintenance and rejuvenation aspects of PK. Having visited Nagpur for extended periods of time, he and Eva are quite the tour guides. They often entice us to join them on the various jaunts around the city. Peter is most helpful with the history of various areas and knows much of the local lore as well. He has a dry sense of humor that I quite enjoy. They are respectful of the limits of what I can do because I am in the midst of my first week of the cleanse. They are in their last week of the month, with a rejuvenative focus. Their energy level is quite a bit higher than mine. He often quips about how far they are roaming away from the clinic, knowing that I had a basti recently. Because they are in the restorative phase of the treatment, he no longer is receiving basti as part of his daily regimen.

On one of our jaunts around the city, I see how Eva has spent her time. She is much quieter than her husband. She has a creative part of herself that emerges through the pictures she takes. She is ever respectful of the people and their children. She always asks first before she takes these pictures. Then she turns around to share the picture on her camera with them. She finds delight in sharing, as do the people she has just photographed. She also has enjoyed drawing. She has done a drawing of the clinic with its various floors and activities. It is hanging in the foyer of the clinic on the bulletin board.

The Tiffins

At lunchtime, they serve the food in tiffins. I am amazed how hungry I am. Yvette from France shares that she is about to go up to the rooftop lounge. I take my tiffin and walk up with her to share the meal. She has been busy doing her laundry for her trip home in two days. I grab my laundry as well, since finding time and getting the only machine available are hard to make happen in the same moment.

As we eat, I discover a vegetable I recognize! It is zucchini. While here, I have seen quite a few vegetables native to India that I have never eaten before. One type of spinach has a more pointed leaf than the spinach in the States. It has a peppery flavor to it. Roti, dal, and rice are the treasures in the tiffin today.

As Yvette finishes her lunch, she hangs her laundry around the perimeter of the upstairs terrace area. The breeze is quite nice today. She comments, "The clothes will dry quickly today!" I agree. She offers to take my tiffin as I want to start my laundry.

We wash our own tiffins so I ask her to simply place my tiffin on the counter. Thanking her, I inform her, "I will clean it when I come back downstairs."

The laundry machine is a two-part system that appears complicated to manage, yet is not once you understand certain steps. But key to the operation is to turn on the electricity via the switch on the wall to the left of the machine. I didn't do so one day, convinced that the machine was broken. Mukul was kind and patient enough to review what was "wrong" with the machine. I had no further problems with the machine after that.

The left side is the washing side of it, where I turn on the water, and as water trickles in, I turn on the timer, arranging for some agitation of water in a deep basin. Then manually, I turn the knob to have the water drain from this side. I fill the basin again with fresh water. I hand rinse the clothes. There is an agitator only on the left side. The right side of the machine is more effective for spinning, or so I find out after the first time I finish washing my clothes. After it feels that the soap is rinsed out sufficiently, I switch the clothes to the right side of the machine. The basin is not as deep. I add the water to this side by turning the knob. Then with the timer set, the basin spins for the allotted time. Finally, the clothes are ready to be hung up and there is room to do so on the clotheslines. I feel the breeze. It remains strong so I know the clothes will dry within the next hour to two. I am happy to have clean clothes.

PASSAGE TO INDIA

My Attire

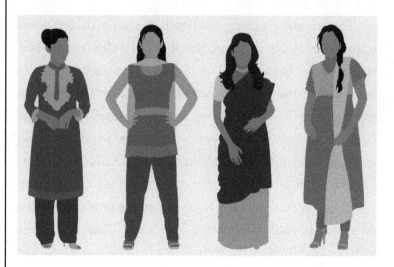

Salwar Kameez

I usually wear *punjabis* or *salwar kameez* while I am in India. These clothes are the traditional attire for women as well as men. Salwar are trousers that are wide at the top but narrow at the ankle. The kameez is a long tunic with various colors, depending on the region of India. I find this style of clothing to be very comfortable and modest enough to meet the standards that India has for how women dress, even foreigners. These cotton clothes are great in the heat as well. And as I only have two or three outfits, I need to wash them to have them ready for the next time I need them.

Today they gave the first shirodhara in the afternoon.

I rested afterward. Yes, there is a lot of down time, but because of the schedule of the bodywork in the morning, with a possible shirodhara later in the day, free time is chopped up quite a bit. If I need a consult with Sunil Joshi or blood work, I do this during free time.

During the cleanse, no spices are allowed. Once the cleanse is over, some spicy options can be considered but it depends on your constitution/dosha. For me, due to my pitta nature, limited spiciness is recommended.

Food and its quality is most important. Warmed, cooked food is preferred. Adding olive oil or ghee (clarified butter) into the cooking process is most important to the diet. These are healthy oils that further support the body.

No leftovers are recommended as the food is considered old and dead and thus not able to nourish the body. The fresher, the better; the closer to the source, the better; homemade is the best, as is having your meal prepared by those who love you.

Dinner soon follows. I am hungry and relish the rice, vegetables, and dal along with the *chapati* (also known as *roti*). The camaraderie of the group is palpable, yet they are welcoming to the three of us who are the last of the group to join for this session of panchakarma. Peter spoke sadly of the time coming to a close. "This has been most restorative for me, and now we are enjoying the rejuvenation treatments, but we leave in three days. It saddens my heart to have to go. It feels so welcoming here. And I have found the PK to be most beneficial in reducing my risk of diabetes. My blood sugars are back to normal. And yes, I watch my diet and sugar intake, but I know that the PK has aided in my return to health. The herbs that Dr. Joshi has prescribed have also helped me."

FOOD AS MEDICINE

Chapati/Roti

Chapati is the daily bread made in many Indian homes. It is used to help pick up the food from the plate. It does not have yeast, is often made with atta flour—a local whole-wheat flour—and it is eaten fresh with melted ghee. Chapatis do not reheat well. They can be made of teff, an ancient grain that is offered in the clinic for those sensitive to wheat or who have diabetes.

I asked about why we were the last of the group this time. Peter explained that the heat in India is the most extreme from March until the monsoons come in June or July. Because of the high temperatures at this time of year, which can reach more than 110 degrees Fahrenheit, most Westerners choose not to come to India or to the clinic. As a result of this, the clinic is closed for extended periods of time through these months until the monsoon season starts. Then, with the rains, it is a little cooler in Nagpur and the clinic may open again. Certainly, it is open in early September. Trainings for ayurvedic technicians happen in August at the clinic.

After more conversation and ginger tea, I am blissfully off to my room. Tired and most ready to go to sleep, I remember to take my herbs. I decide to check emails, as it is morning in the time zone back home. My heart brightens as I see an email from my daughter. All is well! I email her back, sharing a little of the day and about the people I have met. I also see an email from my office that I respond to easily. News from the office has been minimal while I have been here so far. It has taken a lot of preparation to come over to India and it appears that the steps I have taken were sufficient.

I prepare for bed. The night air is cool. I keep the window on the second floor open for some fresh air. I do not need the fan on in the room tonight. As I recline on the bed, I attempt to read the novel I brought but am unable to sustain attention to the plot. I put the book down. Sleep comes swiftly.

Chapter Three

Roller Coaster

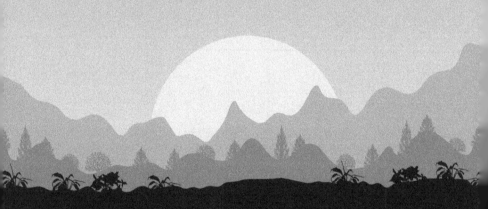

DARK NIGHT OF THE SOUL
MIND ALERT, CHANTING, PRAYING
BODY FATIGUED, SORE

DAY THREE

I had a rocky start this morning. I slept much less than the previous nights. We all retired to our rooms by 9 p.m. or so. Electronics have been recommended to be kept to a minimum, with wi-fi not available in the rooms. Our hosts have requested that we read very little to really take time off from stimulating the brain and our senses. Because of the intensity of the bodywork being done, I am often exhausted at the end of the day. Falling asleep early has not been uncommon. Some nights I forget my herbs. Yet, after four hours of solid sleep, I was up every two hours thereafter with my eyes wide open at 4 a.m. My mind was quite active. Many thoughts tumbled over themselves, about what brought me to this place so far away from home. I wondered what desire led me here. Though I knew what it was, doubts crept in. Feeling very vulnerable in that moment, I chose to chant mantras to calm my mind. Simply saying *"om"* felt very supportive. Also, repeating *"shrim"* helped. My lower back was in pain. Finding a comfortable position in the twin bed was not happening for me, yet I fell asleep at last with the soothing mantras.

I welcomed the morning light. Though tired, I began the ablutions. I noticed that my back was no longer sore after simple stretches. I felt emotionally raw and tender. It felt like I went through the ringer last night. As I reflected on the events of the night, I held a sense of ongoing vulnerability and heart pain. I felt that I was being presented with an inventory of sorts. Having been of service most of my life, I have had little time for receiving the kindness and support that I offer to others. I realized that is something I wanted to change within myself. This idea of accepting the love and kindness of others to further support me...I love the feeling, the medicine, as I sense the resonance of what that would offer. To proceed with my life and ask others to be present in the creation of what I next imagine is what I desire most.

Morning Rituals

On this morning, I review emails from back home. It is early evening in New Mexico. Then it is time for yoga. Each day Pritti presents a slight change from the previous day. She has us practice *pranayama* for a longer period of time. One method she shares with us is to use the phrase "Shri Ram, Jai Ram, Jai Jai Ram" to help with breath control in alternate-nostril breathing. I find it slows my breath down, which allows me to more fully benefit from the pranayama. We practice then stop to notice the benefits to the body and mind. I feel calmer and more settled.

I had known that at some point during panchakarma, it was likely that the emotional roller coaster would present itself. Entering the treatment room on this third day, I disrobe and place myself on the table facedown into the face cradle. As Pravin asks how I'm feeling, suddenly tears start to flow. A tremendous sadness comes over me. I cry as the massage continues. No words can describe the sensation, other than profound ache in my heart. No particular memory, other than what I remember upon arising, comes up for me. It is simply time for release. By the time I need to turn over on my back for that phase of the bodywork, I feel the emotional release has lifted a weight off my shoulders. It seems complete for now.

This is common. A release can simply entail crying spontaneously when you are lying face down. Or someone sharing information with you that is not particularly provocative yet which causes you to feel a sudden sensitivity that you have not noticed before. Layers can be exposed as the week progresses and the bodywork, as well as other interventions, strips away the protected parts of self.

TENDER LOVING CARE

Emotional Releases

These emotional releases are just that—another form of release of the body and brain. Many people find that documenting when and what might emerge from these moments can have some meaning at the time and later. Writing down your thoughts and feelings as well as your emotions may be an option for you.

Yet during this process, simply witnessing what is happening is best. Letting go applies here as well. Just as there is the obvious letting go of the physical toxins through these various modalities, there is also the letting go of emotional toxins. And you can have very good moments as well where you feel very blissed-out and on top of the world.

Having some awareness of what issues have been significant for you can bring insight to the power of PK. As I shared earlier, an unfolding of oneself occurs, and that impacts the chakras. My sense of this is such that, as the person's physical issues are minimized and the body is cleansed deeply, it is then that the chakra cleanse becomes more a part of the picture of PK. I share this from my personal experience and from discussions that I have had with others more versed in the healing art of Ayurveda. For me, this time, there appears to be a cleanse of the heart and throat chakras.

Following the *swedana*, I have a *pinda swedana,* which is a herbed milk bath applied with a herbed rice ball. After that, I am in the steam box for about five minutes. I shower, put on my gown and move to the next room for the neck and lower back basti. I gargle with a warm herbal decoction. As I finish and move back to the massage table, Pravin enters and places the dough carefully, then the warm oil. I had felt a little chill waiting for him but the oils quickly warm me up. He returns in about ten minutes, removing the oil first, then the dough. He leaves some dough on the skin. I will pick or wash it off in the shower. I am spent. I realize I am not interested in talking much at this moment. I get up to go to my room.

I speak to Sunil after lunch. He asks, "How are you doing today?" I share what I notice. He agrees: "Yes, the cleanse can impact you strongly here!" I ask, "What else is the focus for me?" He states, "You have increased *pitta* (the fiery dosha) and disturbed vata (the air dosha*).* We are focusing on reducing the excess fire and calming vata so the strong *kapha* (earth dosha*)* part of you can be more expressed. More cohesion and endurance is then possible!"

"This is very exciting to hear," I said. "I wonder how that is expressed in my body and mind?"

"You experience clarity of thought and senses," he said. "You are more able to express what your heart desires."

Good news for me! I hug him and go upstairs to meditate on all we just discussed, as well as to practice alternate-nostril breathing/pranayama with some gentle yoga.

An Assessment

Each morning before the bodywork starts, we fill out an assessment sheet. It informs both the clinician and the technician how the preparatory phase is going. Questions that are on the form include: When did you take the *tikrita* (medicated) *ghee* and when did your appetite return after taking the ghee? When did you receive the internal basti? How long did you retain the basti? What was the content of the bowel movement expelled? How many bowel movements since the basti was given? This would be the time to share if there are any new physical, mental, or emotional problems or if they have been resolved.

Pravin, the lead ayurvedic technician, and Sunil Joshi review all this information. It is from this form that they make revisions to the daily treatment protocols to adjust to the changes that the person is going through. An example of a change that could happen would be the addition of a basti that may be needed due to back pain a person may be having. Or if there is a limited amount of bowel movements, then the type of internal basti may change to assist with evacuation, which is most necessary during this time.

FOOD AS MEDICINE

Tikrita

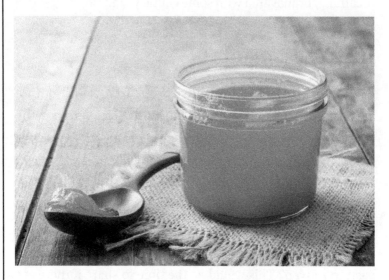

Tikrita, or medicated ghee, contains fifty different herbs.

Tikrita is medicated ghee (clarified butter). It has over fifty different herbs in the mixture. It is given as part of the preparation of the body for the final release on the seventh night. It allows for more toxins to be removed from the body. It also supports the fasting process so you are not so hungry.

The dose is gradually increased depending on your health needs for the week. It is taken upon awakening and at 4 p.m. for seven days; the last dose depends on how well the body has responded to all the various treatments offered during the week as well as your acceptance of what is being offered during this time of intense healing.

I do experience leg cramping one night. They give me extra time for a specific massage for the leg and hip the following day. I do not have any more leg cramps that week.

CELLULAR SHIFT

Restoring Natural Rhythms

Constipation and irritable bowels are significant health issues in the western world. Often this is due to dietary choices, but it can also be medication-related. Most people do not even think about how often they have a bowel movement. It is a good sign of health to have at least one, if not two, bowel movements a day. A morning bowel movement is ideal. We have a natural reflex called the gastrocolic reflex that happens after meals, so it would be most natural to seek to evacuate the bowels after meals.

Today's routine is the same in terms of bodywork as the previous day, except for the addition of a heart basti. I find that particular basti to be very nourishing to the emotional level of my heart. The herbed oil is warm, so it penetrates the skin more easily. I feel it gives me a level of soothing support.

Shirodhara can be done outside of the PK protocol. This is a good thing as its intention is to calm the mind and "pacify" vata, or stress disturbance, in the nervous system. So this procedure adds to the other protocols in reducing the stress the body normally experiences.

I am given a shirodhara today, which is given at the end of the day. I am tired and spent yet feel a sense of inner calm after the release of the emotions at the start of the day.

———

PK allows you to withstand threats and toxins
that diminish you. It has a preventative effect.

———

Pravin comes in to begin the process. I welcome his calming presence. This adds to the overall reverence present in the moment. I find this one of the most blissful procedures known on this planet. I easily move into a deep meditative state and maintain it for the majority of the treatment. I experience moments of silence but also have connected with Divine beings during this time.

I return to my room and meditate. Then I fall asleep.

Nightfall

As darkness falls and the street noise picks up with going-home traffic, I wake up. Taking the third shower of the day, I remove the oil from my hair. Soon it is time for dinner. Neetu has left for the day. We all congregate in the dining hall, reaching for the tiffins. I wonder what is to be served. As I open my tiffin, several of the ten people at the clinic arrive. The rice has cumin today and the spinach is spiced nicely. The dal is warm and tastes almost like split-pea soup. The chapattis are a perfect addition to the meal.

One couple, Sankara and Prema from Chennai, share that their daughter recently married. Prema speaks of the preparation for the four-day ceremony. She smiles easily as she speaks of the happiness of the event. Sankara also is very pleased. And they also welcome the respite that the PK offers to them.

I share the rough night that I have had. One woman shares that she also had been up most of the night. And yet, we both agree that though we are feeling tired in the moment, we feel peaceful at the end of the day. Witnessing what each of us is going through feels good for the moment. Simply sitting with a cup of ginger tea in silence at the end of the evening feels complete for the day.

As I retire to my room, I take herbs for digestion and for support of the brain. I review the day in my journal. My eyelids are closing almost as I am writing. Sleep comes easily.

FOOD AS MEDICINE

Cumin

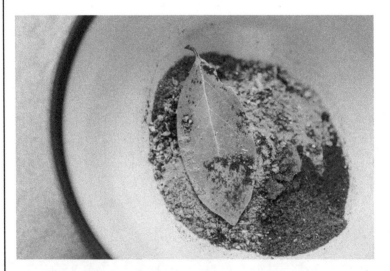

Cumin promotes digestion and improves blood-sugar control and cholesterol.

Cumin seed is a common spice in Indian. It comes from a flowering *Cuminum cyminum* plant in the Apiaceae family. It grows in the Middle East and India. The seed is often used in curries. Health benefits include promoting digestion and aiding in reducing food-borne infections. Research has shown it may help with improving blood-sugar control and cholesterol. It is also rich in iron.

Chapter Four

Bliss

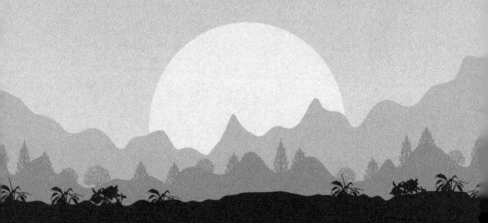

**WARMED OIL TO THIRD EYE
BLISSFUL, SOOTHING, MOST CALMING
WITH SHIRODARA**

DAY FOUR

A thunderclap awakens me in the middle of the night. The rumbling sky keeps me up as the storm rages. Eventually I fall back asleep, and I am up before the alarm, feeling rested. I feel less sore physically as well, and my mind feels really clear today. I hold a sense of awareness and gratitude in my heart. Words flow easily in my journal. Much love fills my heart's center, for myself and for those around me. Accepting love and being cherished is a part of life I am choosing to experience in this moment. The words are simple but profound for me.

Yoga starts a little later today as Pritti had a delay at home. Her daughter needed extra help with her hair before she went to school. Pritti smiled with the wisdom of mother, "There are certain things that only the mother can offer our children!" Hearing this, I see the expectations for the mother here are no different from what we might expect in our own culture. Yet I know that the father in the US is beginning to take on a more of the nurturing role. Pritti and I explore new twists today on the floor. The pranayama with the mantra is a little more difficult to do, but I make a good effort at it. At the end of class, it feels good to move the body with a familiar sequence. I choose to move into *savasana* instead of extended meditation today. It feels good to do so.

Breakfast with some fresh chai is calling me. Neetu serves me a breakfast grain that I am not familiar with, but it appears to be a form of couscous. It is garnished with cilantro. The chai is fresh and warms my heart! I eat alone today. My schedule changes to an earlier time so I finish my meal and prepare to go down for the treatments.

PASSAGE TO INDIA

Hanuman

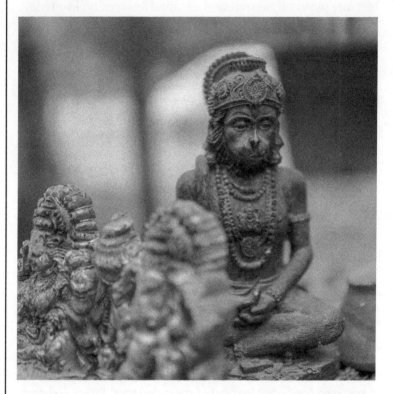

Hanuman, the Hindu monkey god, is shown in devotion to Rama and Sita.

Hanuman, the Hindu monkey god, is a symbol of love, devotion, perseverance, loyalty, and physical strength, as well as service, as he supported the well-being of Ram and Sita in the epic *Ramayama*. This epic inspires you to face life's ordeals and conquer the obstructions presented. Asking for his support can aid in your daily journey to be focused on what matters in your life.

The day feels very fresh outside as I take a walk around the clinic. The clinic comes alive with the rituals of the day. I see the honoring of the guru Bhagwan with the placement of his picture in the foyer. Sankara greets me and walks with me to the Hanuman shrine. The ghee is already burning, as is the incense for Hanuman, who graces a special place near the back of the clinic. Hanuman is the monkey god who serves Ram and Sita. He is seen as a symbol of prana: Without prana, there is no life. Sankara shares, "Hanuman is a symbol of loyalty and calling upon him allows for success in your life. See, he also holds herbs in his left hand that are called to heal." With reverence, Sankara and I stand in silence as we gaze at Hanuman and offer gratitude for his presence at the clinic.

After filling out the daily assessment form, I am aware of how much has shifted in the few days since I have arrived. I feel a calmness that is notably different from the day before. The herbs are assisting me with my digestion. I notice that the simplicity and nourishing aspects of the food I receive each day also support me. With travel, often most of us have problems with constipation due to the lack of routine, creating a vata imbalance. Here, the internal basti and yoga both support me to be as regular as possible.

HEALING OILS

External Basti

External basti are warm, herbal oils placed on the body in areas needing nourishment. This oil can be placed typically over the heart area, lower back or neck area. Placement of the oil is assisted by the positioning of dough that is formed into a circle over the area to be treated. After the dough is securely placed over the area, the oil is poured into the hole created by the dough. One needs to be very still as the jostling of oil can lead to its leaking out. The treatment soothes the area and reduces tension, including muscle tension.

Today's bodywork is the same as the second day. After the shower, I proceed to the next room for the external basti of the day. I see a warm, herbal mixture in a cup near the massage table. Gargling with this is another way the body is prepped, as it further removes toxins and cleanses the throat and mouth. I pick it up and proceed to gargle with it over the sink in the bathroom adjacent to the room. The herbal mixture tastes slightly bitter and astringent. I can handle the taste as it is not in my mouth for very long.

Today is another heart basti. The heart basti is precisely over the heart area. Pravin comes in to place the dough mixture and then the warmed oil into it. It feels very soothing and calming. I remain still for about ten minutes then Pravin enters with his usual smile. He proceeds to empty the oil from the handmade container of sticky dough, then removes the sticky dough. There usually is a little dough for me to remove as well. But before I leave, it is time for the internal basti. Today is a more nourishing oil basti, thus not as stimulating. After it is given to me, I remain still on my back, gently massaging my belly in a counterclockwise manner to aid in the movement of the basti. I sit up, feeling relaxed, yet I have enough energy for what the day may hold.

I welcome the ritual of the bodywork as my body becomes more and more relaxed—and my mind, too—with each successive day. I feel very supported in this environment. I relish the sacredness of the process that presents itself here. I feel deeply honored while the process is happening. Even when I am walking around in the clinic or outside, all are very cordial and happy with their work.

After I am finished for this part of the day, I go upstairs and change into a punjabi. It is time for lunch. The tiffins are all lined up, and I find the one with my name. As I take it, I hear Peter behind me. We had discussed last night, if all works out, that we would be able to go out to explore more of Nagpur on a walk that is part of the daily routine for him and his wife. They have welcomed my presence. I feel strong enough to go now, so after eating our freshly prepared rice, dal, vegetables, and roti, we locate his wife, who is just finishing for the day as well.

FOOD AS MEDICINE

Spicy Food

During a cleanse, no spices are allowed. Once the cleanse is over, some spicy options can be considered but it depends on your constitution/dosha. For me, due to my pitta nature, I limit spiciness in my diet.

The quality of the food is most important. Warmed, not raw, food is preferred. Adding olive oil or ghee (clarified butter) during cooking is beneficial because these are healthy oils that further support the body.

I am most pleased, as I have enough time and energy to go for an extended walk in the city with Peter and Eva. I had the more nourishing basti today, so I am not as worried about walking around the city. One constant challenge in India is finding adequate, hygienic facilities, especially for women. There is no local McDonald's as yet. Everywhere I go around the world,

McDonald's always have reliable and clean bathrooms. It is a most interesting irony that cleanliness is important in a place where the food is very processed.

As we walk to the Shiva Temple on the back roads of Nagpur, Peter shares more about his life. I learn that his diabetes scare happened a year earlier and he came soon after for treatments. "My favorite beverage in the evening had been apple juice, and I was very good about drinking it daily," he said. "Until I learned that I had signs of diabetes. I had been seeing Sunil Joshi for consults. After I learned of my condition, I saw him soon after. Hearing the problem that I had, Sunil said that PK would be most beneficial but, of course, dietary changes are most necessary as well. I soon booked a flight to Nagpur and here I am again. My numbers are quite good!"

Many of the local families of Nagpur are now walking with us. The women are dressed in their brightest saris as are their daughters. Each carries an offering to take to the temple. As we near the temple, we see more and more vendors offering for us to purchase coconuts, garlands of flowers, or rice as offerings to the divine. We turn onto the lane to the Shiva Temple, we all realize that getting inside today will not happen. The lines curve around near the beginning of the lane, with one line specific for women and children and one for men. Many stare at us because there are few foreigners here. All are polite and allow us to take pictures. We ask permission if we take close-ups. Of course, sacred cows are part of the scene. This particular temple has a dairy nearby. Part of the sacredness of the cow is that it offers its milk to us. Certain religious sects will not even drink the milk because their believers see that as taking the milk from a holy animal.

PASSAGE TO INDIA

Mahashivratri

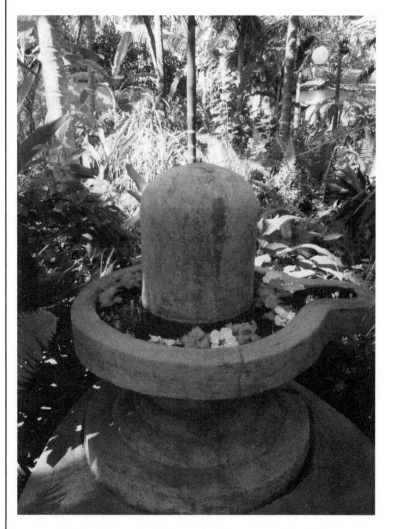

The *linga* is a symbol of the generative energy of the divine.

A special day in the Hindu tradition is the Mahashivratri holiday, a celebration of Lord Shiva, who is seen as the Supreme One, Unmanifest, and of the Trinity, the Creator. He is represented by the *linga*, a symbol of the generative energy of the divine. It is in the shape of a phallus often with a cobra on top which represents the presence of Shakti.

Shakti is the feminine energy of the universe and is what manifests into our world from the Unmanifest. The two are in an eternal dance. One example of their presence in our world would be the sun being Shiva and the sunbeam being the Shakti.

Peter shares with me the importance of visiting the temple for those in attendance today. "Shiva is seen as the most perfect husband. Blessings are sought from him today for those in need and seeking to manifest in their life."

He adds, "Nearby is another temple that we can visit as it will not be as crowded. It is the Hanuman Temple." We walk over there and are able to proceed as the crowd clearly was focused on seeing Shiva today. We spent time in the temple with Hanuman present as well as each of the trinity and their consorts. Eva rings the bell after giving a small donation. The bell aids in taking your wish to the deity.

Now, I am ready to return to the clinic. It is quite warm and we have about a thirty to forty-five-minute walk back to the clinic. I also have a shirodhara procedure happening soon. As we walk back, more cows greet us. They roam the street looking for food. Most look benign, but occasionally a cow can look more fierce. I make room for them whenever I see them. Suddenly, I hear a squeal in the distance. We see pigs in a cluster nearby, free to roam the streets as well.

Back at the clinic, I receive the shirodhara, which is given at the end of the day. Moist cotton balls are placed over my eyes to both reduce stimulation and protect the eyes from the oil being poured over the forehead. I feel tired and spent, yet carry a sense of inner calm after the release of the emotions at the start of the day. My mind is less engaged thus I find I am able to let go of the thoughts as they arise. Floating...that's the word that comes to mind to describe the experience as I am reclining on the massage table.

PK has a rejuvenative effect on the body and the brain. When toxins are reduced, the natural healing of the body can be re-established.

For the shirodhara, Pravin pours warm sesame oil on my forehead for about twenty minutes. It pacifies or quiets vata imbalances, specifically the *prana vayu*. This procedure calms the nervous system down. Often this procedure is done after PK to further maintain the level of cleanse.

Today, I feel the presence of Hanuman and sense the Christ consciousness as well, in my heart and all around me. This shift and connection with the Divine has been facilitated by this and the other procedures via PK. And this deeper way of being with the Divine is what I have been longing for. With this specific treatment, I have had experiences so deep that I have lost the boundaries of my body and feel myself entering a very blissful state. It is only when the dripping of the oil ceases and my head is lifted to scrape the oil from the table that I enter into the room with conscious awareness of my body again.

After the *shirodhara*, I remain on the massage table for five to ten minutes. Or, so I think as I am so relaxed at this point, time has little meaning. When I do finally sit up, I keep the towel that has been wrapped over my head and hair. I then migrate up to my room. I remember to take my tikrita ghee. I keep the oil in my hair for about an hour and sit quietly in meditation. Reducing any stimulation at this point feels really good. I recline after the meditation, taking a deep, restful nap.

I wake to horns honking. As night falls, the air is full of these sounds as vehicles seek to clear the intersection without stopping. Outside, traffic swells. I sit up, feeling a little disoriented. Oh yes, I am in India. The richness of my experience at the temples today lingers. My senses were stimulated maybe a bit more than is good at this time. Maybe not. Being in the community during a festive time enlightens me about the Hindu culture and the people in Nagpur. I find it heartwarming to see families celebrating together. This afternoon, I loved seeing the warm smiles of those standing in line. The experience added one more way to love the charm of India.

I have my third shower of the day to remove the oil from my hair. As I prepare to dress, I check in with how I am feeling. I feel more settled. There is a calm present deep within me. I like this feeling, and would welcome it every day.

Neetu has come again to prepare our meals. As she prepares to leave, I come into the kitchen. It is a long day for her. I smile and say, "Thank you again for the wonderful food you prepare each day for us." She nods her head and smiles. "You're welcome!"

All of us gather briefly to eat our last meal of the day together. I see a few are rushing through their meal. I ask, "What is happening that you are in such a hurry?" I hear from Peter that he had read in the paper that a great pundit (master) playing the sitar in the raga tradition was presenting a concert at 7:30 p.m.

He asks, "Do you want to join us?" I decline. "My day has been full enough and I am feeling too tired to go."

The three of us that are in the midst of PK chose to stay behind. It is a wise decision, as I learn later that the concert goes quite late. As we finish our meals, we sit quietly. After the group leaves, the energy is much more subdued. One person admits he has been working on his computer, though he knows it is best not to do so during this time. He feels inspired by the PK process. His wife was not happy with him, but as she says, "It is his choice. I would prefer he not work now. This is an important time to simply rest and do very little."

I agree with her, as does he, but he simply grins, "And I chose to work on the computer for now." He shares, "I am fully aware of the impact this may have on the outcome."

What he alludes to is the need to follow the prescription of rest and relaxation during this time. The preparatory time determines the outcome of this eight day process. The capacity for the cleanse to be a complete one is compromised if you do not take care of yourself during this time. This translates to resting often, reading little, and taking a gentle daily walk along with a more measured practice of yoga.

For me, it is so much easier to follow the prescription in India as I do not have the tugs of work that have pulled me away from the process in the US. This may explain why it took almost four PKs before I began to understand the depth of the cleanse. This time here in India is truly a gift I have given myself.

TENDER LOVING CARE

Dinacharya

The daily ritual of taking care of yourself (ablutions) is referred to as *dinacharya*. There are behavioral or lifestyle recommendations that are specific for you. The intent is to gain ideal or optimum health to the best of your ability with these lifestyle changes. The daily routine at the clinic that I have shared, with the exception of the excursions that I have mentioned, allows for the mind and body to be most open to healing and the release of toxins. A variation of this daily routine is recommended at the end of the eight days to help maintain these changes that have happened during panchakarma. This requires a commitment to your health in a manner that touches all aspects of your daily life.

As I listen to the Indian couple bicker in an ever so friendly way, I am aware that each of us can be easily pulled from what is best for us in terms of food choices, work issues, spending time with the right people, or following through on meditative practices. Even in the center where we all are being prepared and monitored in a variety of ways, we are pulled in many directions.

I'm off to bed, as prescribed, by 9:30 p.m. No argument from me. First, I take the herbs along with the liquid herbs. I will miss the Dadim, one of the liquid herbs I have been on for the week, as the flavor is slightly sweet, but tart as well, and made of pomegranate. I journal about the day. I am finding I need to carry it with me at all times, as there is so much being shared with me at various points of the day. I check my email in the hallway outside my room. I see an email from my daughter. She is checking in and shares that the family is doing well. I welcome hearing the news and share about my day and the people I have met. I return to my room. Sleep again comes easily.

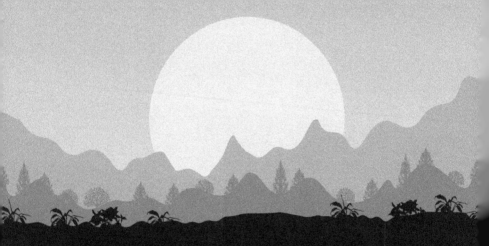

Chapter Five

Going Within

**SENSES WITHDRAWING
FEELING MOST QUIET WITHIN
SEEKING NOW SILENCE**

DAY FIVE

During the night, I feel huge emotional shifts—shifts that significantly impact my sense of self and the importance of cherishing myself at a whole new level. I feel a deepening of the experience from the previous night. I feel a deep love in my heart and tears well up as I touch this sacred and Divine part of myself.

I am able to sleep for almost seven hours, then awaken at 4 a.m. with body pains especially in my left hip area. Moving around does little to ease the discomfort. I end up getting out of bed. After having a bowel movement, my mind calms, and my body too. I am able to find a position in which to continue to rest. Chanting "Om Namah Shivaya" soothes my mind and emotions. This mantra is a way to connect with the Divine within. Later I would share this with Sunil, and he would tell me that the experience reflects the rhythm of the body as it is releasing layers no longer needed, thus purging through ayurvedic principles. Yes, I was releasing toxins with a bowel movement at 4 a.m., and it had ramifications throughout my body and being as, really, there *is no* separation.

HOW IT WORKS

Chanting Mantras

As I have explored the power of chanting mantras, I have learned the power of seed sounds. Known as *bijas* in Sanskrit, they possess the power of sound being amplified into your being. All sacred languages carry the power for us to have this experience. All the mystical lineages of the religions of the world have awareness of this power. Hindu tradition, among others, has brought it into daily life. For me, the power is in the exposure to the mantra, both in listening to them and repeating them out loud as well as silently.

As the morning light enters the room, I arise, feeling calm and rested. What I keep noticing is that the pains and discomfort of the night are gone. I am truly amazed and grateful. I begin the morning routine: shower, morning herbs and decoctions, and morning dose of medicated ghee. I realize that I need to pay attention to the dosing of the *tiktaghrita* (medicated ghee) as I am increasing it significantly. I had forgotten to wait for the hunger to return yesterday. The dosing for me is as follows:

- Day One – ¼ teaspoon morning and 4 p.m.

- Day Two – ½ teaspoon morning and 4 p.m.

- Day Three – ½ teaspoon morning and 1 teaspoon 4 p.m.

- Day Four – 1 teaspoon morning and 4 p.m.

- Day Five – 1½ teaspoon morning and 4 p.m.

- Day Six – 2 teaspoons morning and 4 p.m.

- Day Seven – 2 teaspoons morning, with the second dose determined by Dr. Joshi after an assessment.

I keep thinking I will experience nausea as I increase the ghee, but I never do. It agrees with me in a surprising way.

FOOD AS MEDICINE

Ginger Tea

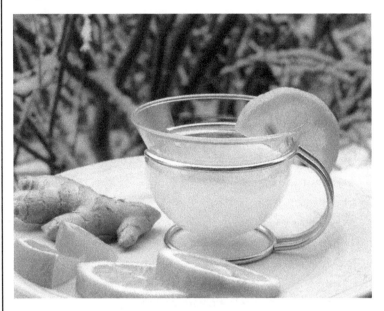

Ginger supports the releasing and healing process—and it reduces nausea.

Ginger is a root herb with many culinary and healing aspects. It is to be consumed daily with ground herbs specific to your dosha needs at the time of the consultation. It is offered throughout the panchakarma week. It supports the releasing and healing process including by reducing nausea. It is recommended as a part of the new daily ritual upon returning home.

After I dress, I have a cup of cool ginger tea. I sit quietly and offer brief prayers for the day, including gratitude for the way my body, emotions, and mind move through the challenges of the night to a place of balance and calm in the morning.

YOGA SPOTLIGHT

Personalizing Your Yoga Practice

A new evolution in yoga explores ways for it to be therapeutic and accessible for those with limitations. Chair yoga, for instance, is great for those who cannot get to the floor. Most postures can be modified to be supportive of your health challenges. Benefits truly can be gained with these modifications. Many yoga studios will offer specific classes for those with back issues as well as other health issues.

Trauma-informed yoga is a way to approach trauma issues without having to talk about it. The release of feelings and emotions on the yoga mat or in the chair can happen regardless and are left there. There is no need to discuss it if you have no desire to do so.

Restorative yoga is one example of how yoga can assist in calming the body and mind. This form of yoga allows for positions to be held for up to five minutes in reclining positions with props to support the body. Use bolsters or blankets as well as other props to maximize the support you need, which aids in calming body and brain.

This morning's yoga session is almost crowded. I realize that several members of the group are leaving later today. Eva confides that she wanted to experience the session with Pritti one last time. It feels good to move the body. The pace and the postures include twists to aid in the digestion and further detox the body. Pritti offers modifications as needed. The age range in the room is from forty to seventy-three, many of us with various ailments including knee and hip issues. We work on a tile floor with little padding, so each of us uses a blanket or another yoga mat.

We practice pranayama techniques included kapalabhati breathing, which I find invigorating. Then we practice a seated meditation. I find my mind to be a little restless today and need to focus on a simple mantra and breath more than usual. After a brief savasana, we finish the session. I can feel the nice release that yoga provided.

Breakfast is calling. The aroma of the savory herbs fills the yoga room, which is next to the kitchen. A warm, fragrant cup of chai is waiting as I walk in to see Neetu pouring it into a mug, wearing her usual bright smile. I ask how she is and she nods, "Good! And you?"

I share, "So much better than yesterday!" I thank her for the chai. I really enjoy the morning time and chat with the others as they arrive for breakfast as well. I note anticipation as well as sadness in the air. The majority of the group leave today to return to their respective countries.

This includes Peter and Eva, who are returning to Switzerland. I share that I will miss them. They enjoy walking as much as I do! Peter has been an incredible ambassador, sharing the parts of Nagpur I would not have known to explore. He helped me to locate my favorite place in town to find the best CDs that India had to offer. It was a mini Best Buy of sorts, but you never would know it as we walked up to it, because the storefront blends in with the others and the signage indicates electronics. Another gem was the local farmers' market tucked away from the main street near the clinic. I have scheduled two free days after the finish of PK, and I make a mental note that I want to be able to eat fruit that peels before I continue on to New Delhi. I look forward to enjoying a banana, as fruit is not part of the diet during the eight days of PK at the clinic.

Apparently, the cleanse is better without the fruit, as people have fewer issues with bloating and gas.

Encountering India

The day before they leave, Pierre, Eva, and I explored the Indian version of a supermarket, which is quite tiny by our US standards. I had noticed security was tight. When we entered, I was asked to leave my bags in the front with the security person and given a container in which to put items that I want to purchase. Then I passed through the turnstile. That day, Pierre and Eva were on a mission to stock up on Himalaya-brand bath and beauty products because they are very cheap in India; not so in Switzerland. The price listed on the package includes tax, so they know the cost before arriving to the checkout counter. I noticed the haphazard way the shelves were stocked, with the products not lined up well and easily falling to the floor. Someone was stocking the shelf, and I observed he was making a sincere effort but still seemed unclear about how to be more effective. I went off to explore other aisles. I did not see much fresh produce, but then I realized most people simply go to the outdoor market for that. Instead, I saw lots of processed, salty packages of potato chips or chickpeas. Lays potato chips have a strong presence in India. It appears that since I was last in India two years ago, the amount of processed food available to Indians has increased. That includes the takeaway options rather than home-cooked meals available in various lodgings, as I learn later in New Delhi. This saddens me, as the quality of the food is never as good as home-cooked, and you don't know how fresh the delivered food actually is.

Unlike in the States, as we headed to the checkout someone added up the tab and presented a total on a slip of paper. I handed that to someone else, who took my payment and put the items in a plastic bag. Then the clerk handed me the bag. I walked through the turnstile to the guard, who requested evidence of final sale and inspected my bag. By the time I left the store, three individuals had touched the products I had purchased. India is excellent about creating layers of work for the people. There can be inefficiency with this approach, but it certainly keeps people employed.

The day after the Shiva holiday, Pierre, Eva, and I had also gone to other temples, both of them Shiva temples, both of them nearly empty—quite a contrast to the day when it was standing room only. The larger temple had many beautiful deities in various areas of the grounds.

CHAKRA FOCUS

Ganesha and the Root Chakra

Ganesha, known as the remover of obstacles, aids us in feeling grounded. Our first chakra, the root or muladhara chakra, has the symbol of the elephant. Ganesha is one of the deities supporting this root chakra.

A larger Ganesha temple in Nagpur is located on top of a hill in the city, and small ones exist in various neighborhoods. We have one close to the clinic in Nagpur, and I often stop there to pay homage to Ganesha and Hanuman. When I was last there, the caretaker and Hindu priest recognized me and recalled I was from Albuquerque. This was a nice surprise.

Across the street is another smaller temple near a roundabout. It was busy with visitors paying homage to Shiva as well as other deities. The bell that hung over where you stand to offer prayer was rung often. That day I decided to break off from Pierre and Eva to find CDs I wanted to buy.

As I bade them goodbye, I walked down the side of the street, instead of the sidewalk. In India, sidewalks are not in best repair, and often vendors have extended their store onto the sidewalk. Also, the height of the sidewalk can be quite high in contrast to the street. The monsoon season brings lots of rain and flooding. The end result is most people walk on the street along with cars, motorbikes, and bicycles. And of course, the occasional cow as well as stray dogs. The cars employ the British style of driving, so I practice looking in the opposite direction. Hesitation is not your friend in India. Being careful is necessary, but walking with an air of confidence works best.

On my mission, I was successful: I found the CDs I had been told about in the clinic. The store I found had a whole wall of CDs to choose from, with the option to listen to them in the store. But I did not need to do that: I knew which one I wanted to buy. The clinic plays certain CDs during the treatments. I had found one that was light and upbeat.

Pleased with my newfound treasure, I started my walk home. Heading down the street to the clinic, I heard my name called. I turned and saw Sunil's nephew, Gaurang, flagging me down from his scooter. I waved at him. "Do you want a ride?" he asked.

I said, "Sure! I am hot and thirsty!" The street was busy with going-home traffic at that hour.

He pointed to the back seat and said, "Jump on!" I was ever so happy to have a ride home.

At the clinic, he dropped me off and I turned to him, "When will I see you to catch up?"

He promised to visit later in the week. He waved at me and said, "I will!" We had met on a trip to India four years prior and with the connection via Facebook, we have stayed in touch. In fact, he is a good photographer and shares his pictures.

Entering the Quiet

I start the bodywork again bright and early. It is a full day. I am feeling emotionally strong today, and my body feels strong, too. My body is becoming one very well-oiled body. I notice that I feel very quiet. I do not chat with Pravin and Raju as before. They work quietly, respectful of my need to be present within. I notice the aromas of the oils, the sounds of the room with a CD of a Ganesha mantra in the background, along with the steam hissing from the pot, the touch of the hands of these experienced bodyworkers only going so deep and in sync with each other. Other days, I have noticed these sensations, but with my chatting, I did not sense them as today. I feel a tenderness, a rawness with my emotions. And a need to keep them close to me. No sharing of words for me today.

We start with the two person abhyanga, followed by the steaming process for the skin (swedana) along with *nasya* oil in the nose. Today is another *pinda swedana*, followed by the steam box. The sadness persists. I take the requisite shower, noticing how amazingly soft my skin is after this last series, and the hot water adds to the more relaxed feeling in my body. I wrap myself in a gown and proceed to the next room. As there is more oil to be applied, I do not dress in the clothes that I wore into the session just yet.

It is basti time. But first, I gargle with a warm, herbal mixture of triphala. Today, Pravin gives the neck and lower back basti. He is ever so diligent in placing the handmade dough in the prescribed area, and then places the warm oil. It feels very soothing. I am able to be still enough today without spilling any of the contents. I am pleased with myself having accomplished this simple maneuver. My thoughts focus on checking in with my body and noticing that tightness in one hip persists at the oddest times. Especially in the present position. The bolster under my knees relieves the pressure enough that I relax. The sadness feels connected to my awareness of the people leaving here again, yet I know from previous PKs that there is more below the surface. Simply observing my feelings and not getting too attached to them is an important strategy for me now and in my daily life beyond PK.

———

With PK, you can release stuck emotions, especially the toxic ones. As toxic emotions bubble to the surface, witness and release them in the moment as they appear.

———

After the external basti, Pravin siphons out the oil then removes the dough. Now it is time for the internal basti, which is oil-based. Pravin administers the basti very easily, gently. He reminds me to rest on my back for a few minutes. I rest on my back for the requisite time, actively rotating my hands counterclockwise on my abdomen. There is some gurgling coming from the abdomen, but otherwise I do not feel any pressure. I sit up and take off the gown to put on the clothes I wore down to the clinic.

Back in my room, I see it is close to noon. I walk to the kitchen and see that most of the meal is almost ready. As always, it is good to see Neetu. I greet her, "How are you since I last saw you at breakfast?" She nods her head from side to side, "All is good." She is finishing filling the tiffins. I pick mine up and carry it to the table. She shares, "I have two children at home, my husband and his mother. I now go home to cook for them!" She is always on the move during the season when the clinic is open.

TENDER LOVING CARE

Reverence for the Food We Eat

Gratitude is so important at all levels of our lives but ever so important with the food we eat. It is important to have some awareness of who has prepared the food, as well as the intention of the person preparing the food. Prayer over our food is a step in that direction, as the energetics of the prayer assists in allowing the food to assimilate into our body much more easily. I recall readings from Neil Douglas-Kloss I found once when preparing for a workshop I presented which explored how blessing our food was seen as an ancient way to raise the energetics of the food to support us better.

At lunch, it is very quiet as those who are leaving are out buying last-minute items for the trip home. I eat mindfully. Enjoying each bite without talking takes on another quality of being present with the food before me...it is nourishing me at so many levels. Simply put, the physical aspects of eating are pretty clear, but it is the other levels that are equally important but rarely noticed or talked about. This includes the love and attention that Neetu puts into the food at the emotional level. The prayer I said over my food before I started to eat further supports the nourishment I receive at the Spirit level.

This afternoon, I decide to stay in the clinic during my free time, except for a brief jaunt to a folk arts festival with Alberto, who is from Italy. He had not spoken much to me when the others were around, but as they are soon to be gone, he begins to share more. The folk festival had been rained-out the day before, and he needs to purchase gifts for his family back home. So I say, "I need to purchase some gifts as well. I will go with you."

At the festival, we find a tent with handiware from Kashmir. The vendor convinces us that he has the best deals and hands us a card, inviting us to Kashmir. He is quick to share that the state is a safe place to visit. I recall that not to be the case but do not argue with him. Kashmir is near the border of Pakistan and Afghanistan, and there have been conflicts that have spilled into the state at times. There are often travel advisories given for that part of India.

PASSAGE TO INDIA

Folk Art Festival

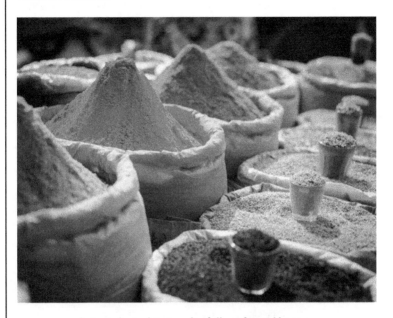

January brought a ten-day folk art fair to Nagpur.

Near the clinic, there is a fairground with several standing buildings reflecting the diversity of folk art in India. During January, there is a ten-day fair that brings many to share their wares. There is artisan furniture, jewelry, shoes, stone carvings, and textiles including clothing and pashmina shawls. Also vital are the supplies for puja, the daily cleansing ceremony performed at home or at temple. Bargaining is expected as prices typically are not set. Then, each evening of the festival, there are musical groups that reflect the breadth of India in song, costume, and dance.

Alberto is pleased with the pashmina scarves. I see colors that may please my mother and sisters, maybe my daughter. I pick several colors and bargain with the vendor to reduce the price.

It works! Then again, I do not bicker too much. I recall the last time I was in India that the woman I was with would drive a much harder bargain. She would walk away if not happy with the price drop. I have a deep red pashmina shawl that she bargained for me. I treasure that shawl and often travel with it.

Alberto and I return to the clinic in the same taxi. Alberto had bargained with the taxi driver to stay for the time we were shopping because the festival is a little off the beaten track. The last time Alberto went, he could not find a taxi to return to the clinic. I am glad Alberto knew how to plan this time.

I have time to rest before the shirodhara. After I have rested, I remember to take the ghee at 4 p.m. I usually have the hardest time remembering to take it then. I want to take it early enough so that I will have an appetite for dinner. As the dose increases each day, it takes longer for my appetite to return.

I walk down the stairs and wait in the foyer. The local paper is available to read. I review the stories. India is facing a huge election this year, and the favorite, Modi, is loved by the people of India because of his humble roots. The pages are filled with discourse about the candidate's strengths and weaknesses. Most of the Indians I have spoken with about him welcome him running for office.

It is time for the shirodhara, time to put worldly thoughts about politics and life aside for now. Pravin escorts me to the room and we share a little about the day. I ask about his family and hear that his son and wife are well. I am supine on the massage table. Pravin starts the dripping of the oil. It is just warm enough. I feel my mind letting go of the thoughts of the day. I am present with the sensations of the oil over my forehead. Pravin creates a gentle rhythm as he moves the oil back and forth. I quickly grow quiet. Conversation is not recommended. As I relax more and more, I move to an interior place. No longer noticing the external sounds of the room or beyond, I am aware of my breathing as it gradually deepens. Then I lose track of my breath as well. I almost fall asleep this time, but Pravin clears his throat quietly. It is enough to bring me back into the room. He finishes and removes the excess oil from my hair and the table. After wrapping my hair in a towel, he leaves the room in silence, as I know what to do. I remain still for a few more minutes. I sit up and feel a little lightheaded. I stay seated a little longer.

Returning to my room, I continue being quiet. I decide to rest today, instead of meditating, as I feel the need to do so.

Night falls at 6 p.m. always here in India because it is close to the equator. I sit up from my brief nap. The oil has been in my hair long enough. I shower. Dressing for dinner, I notice that I have a level of inertia that is uncommon for me. I typically am on the go, but now I feel the need to be present and quiet. I like the feeling for now. I know that I appreciate the energy that I usually have to get things done. For now, being present in this way feels good.

As I arrive for dinner, I hear the voices of the East-Indian couples in the kitchen. I take my tiffin and sit down to listen. The older couple have been in their room most of the week. The husband brings the meals to his wife as her knee pain has been intense, but she has been feeling better so is eating in the communal dining area of the kitchen tonight. She wears a saffron-colored sari tonight. She has very thick white hair that is very long and she usually wears it in a bun. She has let it down tonight, and she is very animated. I turn to Sankara and ask him, "Could you please translate?" because the wife does not speak English. Through Sankara I hear about the incredible healing journey the wife has had in the past six months, which is when she began to come consistently to the ayurvedic clinic. The wife is able to ambulate now, where before the pain and the arthritis was too intense for her to move very much. She can also have periods of time with little to no pain.

She then shares with a huge smile, "I have been healed in part because of the love I feel from those treating me here. They should change the name and add 'prema' [meaning love] to the name of the clinic." We all smiled. And we agreed!

After the five of us bid our good nights, my heart is resonating with her. I have felt the love and the appreciation of the staff throughout the week. That is part of the draw for me to keep coming back. I prepare for bed, feeling much gratitude in my heart.

Chapter Six

Sweet Clarity

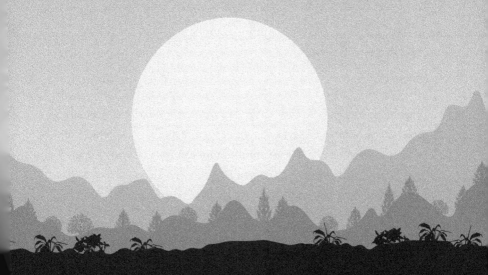

SENSES WITHDRAWING
FEELING QUIET WITHIN ME
PREFERRING SILENCE

DAY SIX

On this day, at this phase, I encounter something unique to the week—PK brain. Though not an official term, the name is an attempt to describe what many have noticed about PK. The deepening of the process and its impact on the senses is referred to in this way. PK brain refers to the sense of being less in touch with the external world, more focused internally. You can be a bit goofy and preoccupied during this phase. It is important to have supportive people around at this time. If not, your own company may be the best for the time being. Be gentle with yourself, with a focus on self-care between the bodywork sessions. That may be all you can do.

HOW IT WORKS

PK Brain

This is a colloquial term that references the state of mind that happens around day five. You feel a bit disconnected from the world around you. You may feel a bit ungrounded and emotionally fragile. There can be an internal focus with a need to be quiet. Time feels irrelevant and the worries you have had seem to melt away. Being present with what is unfolding is possible.

In the past, I have attempted to work part-time during PK. I have found this harder and harder to do with each subsequent treatment. My personal experience has been that there is a foundation that builds upon itself, so now my body and brain begins to prepare for the cleanse a few days before I even start the formal process. Because of this foundational work, I entered into the state of releasing sooner and deeper than I had the last time I did PK. It appears to me to be a body memory of where I left off from the previous PK. And the body simply moves back to the level it remembers. So for each subsequent PK, it moves me deeper and deeper into the process. It is hard to take part in my work as a psychiatrist and be fully present for the depth of internal shifting with PK simultaneously. When I stay in Albuquerque and do a PK week, it is hard for me to completely take time off work. Hence my desire to go to India. I am off the grid for the most part and truly able to be present for the furthest depth of healing possible. And I find that I reflect on this challenge I have back in Albuquerque every time I am in India for panchakarma. The level of introspection and desire to be quiet only grows as the week progresses. Having the luxury of time to myself is one of the gifts I am giving myself.

This internal state of calm and centeredness is brief at this point but most welcome. I have had longer periods of time with a sense of calm.

As the body heals, so does the brain. You
gain the ability to think with more clarity.

The day started off on a good note in that I finally slept well, with less body discomfort and soreness. The day felt quite humid as it had rained through most of the night. This actually led to reduced street noise in the early morning hours. I awakened a few times but returned to sleep quickly. One time when I woke up, I was aware that I now had a fully opened third eye, my sixth chakra. How this would impact me I was not sure, but I knew I needed to explore this concept.

CHAKRA FOCUS

Chakras Opening Up

Chakras are defined in the ayurvedic tradition as areas of swirling energy near the many endocrine systems in our body. Some say they serve as conduits for energetic transfer into our body and back out again.

We have seven main chakras but there are many smaller ones in various parts of the body. The sixth one is associated with the pineal gland and allows for a certain level of intuition to be present for the person.

I complete my morning ablutions. I remember to write down the times when I had a bowel movement and any other nuances that will be noted on paper later in the day. I take my herbs and the medicated ghee. I dress for yoga. I quickly check emails because it is evening in the United States. Again, no unusual or significant issues to note, but I respond to a few emails from friends and family. (Later I learn that some issues had arisen during my time away, but everyone was careful about including me due to the distance and the fact that I was on sabbatical.)

HOW IT WORKS/PRANAYAMA

Bhastrika

Bhastrika, or bellows breath, is a particular form of breathing that is quick to build heat in the body and can stoke *agni*, which is the "fire in the belly." It is quite energizing. Often done early in the morning. It involves a quick out breath followed by a quick in breath. It is repeated for a minute or so, and is done best with a teacher present, if you are a beginner.

Seetali, or rolled-tongue breath work, is also beneficial. In *seetali*, you breathe slowly through your rolled tongue as if drinking through a straw. This helps to cool the body and brain quickly and can be utilized as a counterbalance if you are overheated from certain breath work or from a vigorous pace in certain yoga asanas. It reduces pitta in the body. It is thought to impact blood pressure, so if you have low blood pressure it is good to be cautious.

With the others gone, only four people come to yoga. Pritti begins each session with the Guru Dev prayer, chanting, "Jai Ram, Shri Ram, Jai Jai Ram." She leads a standing sequence with vinyasa flow. I do shoulder and hip rolls with the movement, starting with the larger joints, moving to the smaller joints. The focus of the pranayama is bhastrika (bellow) breathing followed by alternate-nostril breathing. I feel the ease of how my body is moving today. I notice that the yoga postures/asanas are further reducing tension and tightness in my body and mind. Pritti shows us another pranayama. She tells us, "Roll your tongue. Then seek to breathe through your tongue. This helps to cool off pitta and can help reduce hypertension." I practice this breathing technique. I notice that I am able to sense a bit of coolness, certainly at the tip of my tongue as the airflow moves through there.

Given the option to meditate after this breath work instead of *savasana*, I sit and meditate. It comes easily today with less of the monkey mind present. I can tell that I am quieter internally with fewer thoughts distracting me. Yet, I also am aware of needing to stay in touch with my body during this process. This is why I have found my own daily practice of yoga to be most helpful at home. It keeps me grounded and aware.

Savoring the Experience

At breakfast, Neetu adds cilantro to the breakfast plate she serves me. I have to say I am wishing for those mung-bean pancakes again, but I know that she follows a menu. The chai is quite good this morning, and I decide to have a second cup. Neetu serves me the chai with a smile and shares that Shalmali Joshi has created the menu. I appreciate the wholesomeness as well as the simplicity of the meals. No milk (other than the milk which is fresh daily in the chai) is served, which aids in reduction of mucous production. No fruit is served either, to limit the challenges in PK. At the table, I notice a freshly ground mixture of sesame seeds, mango powder, cumin, turmeric, and salt available for us to use instead of salt and pepper. If you request it, you can get a spicy chutney on the table, but not often, because most of us having PK need to avoid spicy condiments. I find Indian hot spicing to be much more than my palate can handle. This is coming from a person who lives in the land of green and red chiles where the heat/spiciness can vary quite a bit.

FOOD AS MEDICINE

Ginger Tea, with a Twist

Ginger tea is available throughout the day. I enjoy the tea, having several cups a day. At home, I make my own freshly grated ginger tea in the morning and again at night. I have substituted the ginger tea for coffee. In addition to the fresh ginger, there are prescribed herbs that I grind at home. These herbs are given as part of the at home regimen after PK. They can change some, but they are a variation of the following herbs: coriander, fennel, licorice, cinnamon, fenugreek, flax seed, turmeric, and cardamom. For sweeteners (I prefer no sweetener), honey, stevia, or maple syrup are healthy choices. Jaggery, dried sugar cane, is available at the clinic. In the kitchen, filtered water is freely available.

After I finish my meal and clean the one dish and pieces of silverware I used, I prepare for the bodywork for the sixth day. It is different today from the other days. There is no pinda swedana or steam box.

Singing along to the latest mantra that is playing in the room, Pravin comes in to apply the brown herbal oil mixture. He applies this mixture on one side of the body, then I flip over for him to finish the other side. It feels like a good scrub, yet it is a gentle process. I feel really relaxed. And it looks like I am covered in chocolate. After fifteen minutes to allow the paste to dry on my body, I am given a small towel to help with wiping the mixture off my body for when I shower.

In the shower, I notice how soft my skin feels. Afterward, I put on a hospital gown and move to the next room to receive the internal basti. I first gargle with a warm mixture then go to the massage table to have the basti. Pravin comes in and administers it. He asks, "How are you doing now?" I tell him that I feel really good. After I gently rub counterclockwise for a minute or so to help move the fluid from the basti into the descending and transverse colon, I lie quietly for about ten to fifteen minutes as prescribed, feeling very calm and rested.

TENDER LOVING CARE

The Chocolate Treatment

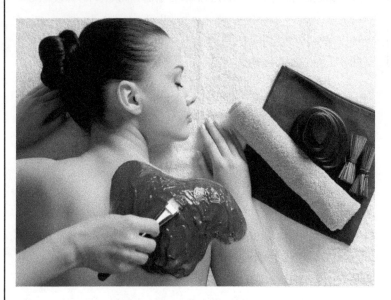

Utsadana, or the chocolate treatment, improves circulation.

This body treatment, *utsadana*, involves application of an oily chocolate-colored herbal mixture to the body. These herbs aid in the reduction of pitta dosha and inflammation in the body. It also improves circulation. Exfoliation is a part of the process as well.

In my room, I take time before lunch. All around me, the clinic is much quieter. After the five of us leave, it will close for a few months. I can feel the energy of the clinic slowing down. I had seen Raju on my way up to my room. "I have not been home in three months!" he said. "I look forward to seeing my family."

The pace of the clinic is such that it is hard to leave, even for a weekend. "That must be really hard for you!" I said.

He shook his head, "It is. But I keep in touch by phone."

Raju stays on site at the clinic and is available if problems arise on the grounds. He is the one who locks up at night and is the first to open the doors in the morning. In addition, there is a security guard outside. Raju also is in charge of the small library on site. I have to catch him at the right time to borrow books because they are locked up in the community room where the yoga is held.

I have a few books from the library. One is an illustrated children's book on the Ramayana. It is colorful and engaging, telling the love story of Sita and Ram and the beloved Ganesha. Ganesha had no awareness of his powers until he wound up leaping over the ocean to help out Ram. It made me wonder about myself and others. We often do not know what strengths we have until tested in certain circumstances. In those moments, those strengths that were dormant come forth.

Sita was also tested, as she was banned for a period of time from where she was living with her husband. She remained faithful during that time, her love for Ram remaining strong.

Soothing My Head

Lunch is served in the tiffins as usual. Today Neetu has prepared okra with a mixture of Indian spices that included mango powder at the end of the sauté, which is the secret to the okra not being sticky. That and not leaving the lid on too long. Today's rice has the aroma of coconut. With the dal and chapati,

Neetu has presented a complete, balanced, and flavorful meal. I am content.

FOOD AS MEDICINE

Mango Chutney

Dried mango chutney is a ground herbal mixture of mango powder, turmeric, cumin, sesame seeds, and salt. This herbal mixture is used to flavor food much as we use salt and pepper in the United States. Mango powder is high in vitamins C, B, D, and B6 along with beta carotenes. It is often used in Indian cooking. Mango chutney is tridoshic, which means all three doshas are able to cook with it or use it as a condiment. It is balancing and supportive.

After I take my afternoon herbs, I walk in the neighborhood, as it is not too hot today. I have completed the shopping I had wanted to do. I remember shopping for readymade clothes at one of the local shops called Fab India with Pierre and Eva. They had displays similar to those in retail clothing stores in the US, and I could pick the clothes that I wanted to try on with minimal help from the retail staff. They were around but not too intrusive. They had a room available to try the clothes on for size. They had a nice range of sizes including slighter larger sizes for Westerners. We are generally taller and larger than the average East Indian. In the more typical Indian stores, I point at what I want and then the staff pull out the item for me to look at and review. Then, as there is no room available to try the clothes on, I have to guess if it will fit. Often the storekeeper will offer advice about size but it still can make for a tough decision.

In the late afternoon, I am given a hair/scalp massage with heated oil, followed by Pravin placing a warm towel over my hair. Pravin then follows this with a face massage with rose cream, then a herbal mask. Once Pravin washes the mask off, he sprays rose water over my face. Now, I feel very relaxed and pampered. No external basti today, only the internal cleansing basti. And no shirodhara today.

I take this afternoon to rest for a period of time and meditate a little. I reflect on the past few days. Already it has been a rich experience on the physical, emotional, mental, and spiritual levels. I have been in India for less than a week yet already feel pretty acclimated to being here again. The time two years ago had been right after the Christmas holiday. That time was for PK alone, and I returned home within two days of finishing the PK. That time the re-entry into my life was most interesting, to say the least. This time I hope that the shifts I experience will be supportive and good for me. This time I will extend my stay to see about further supporting my journey towards spirit (but what happens there will be a story for another time).

The Eve of Virechana

As I go down the hall to dinner, I hear the voices of Sankara and his wife. I greet them with a big smile, "One more day before the virechana! Are you ready?"

They both nod and she shares, "We have been busy! And, yes, God willing all will go well!"

Virechana is a purging procedure that happens on the evening of the seventh day of the cleanse and involves taking herbs at a prescribed time near bedtime to allow for the ama and other toxins to be pulled from the digestive system. The timing is later in the evening to allow for the release of excess pitta from the body during the pitta time of the night. It can make for a long night or a short night, depending on your perspective.

HOW IT WORKS

Virechana

Virechana is a classical PK technique to remove excess pitta from the body via the small and large intestines. It is a purging procedure and is what the first six days of panchakarma prepare you for. If you have had enough preparation, you experience a release of toxins that are pulled from the body via the gut. The prescribed time is determined by nature but aided by a herb taken about two hours before, and again, two and half hours after the meal, which itself has been made to have enough bulk to assist in the process.

As we sit down with our individual tiffins, we each comment on the freshness and quality of the meals. Sankara and his wife also admit that they prefer heavier spicing. Living in the south of India, he notes, "We have our morning coffee, then I go and sit at my computer for hours at a time. She has to remind me when it is time to eat!"

I comment, "I find it hard to believe that you drink coffee in such a hot climate." They reply, "We love coffee and prefer it to chai!"

We chat a little longer then retire to our rooms. It is almost 8:30 p.m. Soon it is bedtime. I make some notes about the day and take the evening herbs. The dadum (pomegranate) elixir is still my favorite! I check in with myself. It feels like a good fatigue with little body discomfort. My mind is pretty mellow for the moment. I even choose to not check my email this time. Plus, I have fashioned a way to be more comfortable on the bed through the night! I again try to read the novel I brought but fall asleep instead.

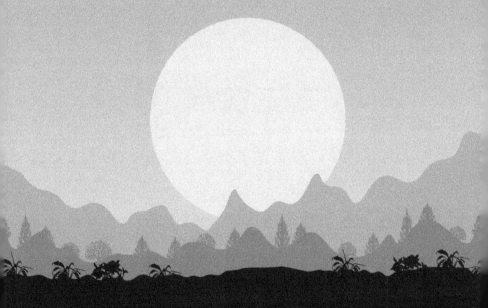

Chapter Seven

Great Expectations

ANTICIPATION

ANXIOUS YET PREPARED, PRESENT

ATTITUDE MATTERS

DAY SEVEN

This is a big day; the day of preparing for *virechana.* The entire week of bodywork and herbs has helped to pave the way for the process to happen easily and safely.

I feel a sense of anticipation. My body feels very relaxed as the night's sleep was restful and refreshing. I wonder if I will be one of those individuals who have not been able to complete the cleanse to the level that is needed to proceed to this last part of the process. It never has happened to me yet. I begin with the daily shower using lots of hot water. I love the hot water and with the solar panels on the rooftop, the clinic never runs out. Given how often we take showers throughout the week, this is a good thing! The ayurvedic soap the clinic provided is thinning considerably. I make a mental note to ask for another bar. Then I scrape my tongue and take my herbs and elixirs. I ingest the medicated ghee, up to two teaspoons now. I am thinking about the day and how it will unfold. Also, emotionally I am feeling pretty settled, with little anxiety. It is a very nice feeling to experience. I sit for a brief period of time and meditate as well as offering prayers for the day.

Yoga is soon to start. I quickly make my bed and put away the clothes in the room. Today is one of the days that the cleaning attendants will sweep and wash the floors in the bathroom and bedroom. They will also change the sheets today.

Yoga begins with just two of us. Pritti moves us through the asanas after sharing the prayer to Guru Dev. We move through the sun salutation, repeating the mantra for the sun with each repetition of the vinyasa offering a different name for it. It is done at a very slow pace. I add the ocean breath with the movement. This breath is performed with a slight constriction in the back of the throat. It also is referred to as the "Darth Vader" breath. Using this breath helps me to keep focused to the moment in the asana.

YOGA SPOTLIGHT

Ujjayi

This breath work is performed by partially closing off your glottis and is done easily as you try to breathe like Darth Vader does in the Star Wars movies. This breath offers many benefits, the main one being to keep you focused and present while doing yoga poses.

Supporting Elimination

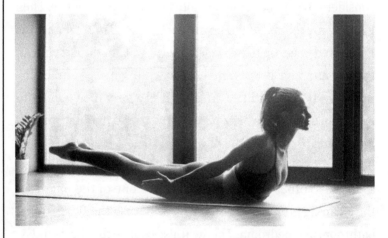

An example of locust pose, for massaging the internal organs.

Gentle twists, seated or lying down, aid in gently squeezing the intestines. Locust pose involves lying face down on the mat. Gently lift your legs up, then your torso with arms extended towards the back of the feet. Both aid in allowing elimination to be more regular.

We move to the floor after finishing the standing poses. I am ready to be on the floor. The focus here is to stretch out the back and the muscles of the legs. Twists are also incorporated daily to support the digestive process. The twists aid in moving the intestines and squeezing them in a gentle way. Elimination is improved when these moves are done regularly. One other pose to aid the body in elimination is the locust pose. We do this pose today as well. I am face down on the mat. Pritti instructs us to raise our shoulders up with our head down initially, bringing our arms down near our body, then to bring up our heads, followed by our legs. I remember to breathe. This posture strengthens the lower back as well. After holding the locust pose briefly, I rest with my head down. I repeat the pose with Pritti's cue. I like this pose and I find it to be a gentle backbend for me.

Pritti teaches another pranayama option today. We start in a seated position. Pritti tells us to simply focus breathing through the left nostril four to five times then the right nostril. We first close off the right nostril to start the sequence, then switch our fingers to the opposite nostril. This process can cool off the body when the focus of the breathing is on the left nostril or energize the body when the breath is just coming in and out of the right nostril. I notice the difference pretty quickly. I am continually amazed at how breath work is so simple to practice yet so profound and immediate in its effect.

I decide to stay seated again to finish the time allotted for practice of yoga for the day. I am able to go quite deep today in the few minutes we are sitting. A deep quiet is present within and I am able to focus on the third eye very easily. It is not always like this! I hear Pritti nearby starting with the Gayatri prayer. It brings me back into the room in the most gentle of ways. I feel my heart moved by the moment. It feels very special and sacred. I approach Pritti and share, "I feel very moved this morning. I am grateful for your presence and offerings today." And then ask for a hug.

Pritti responds, "I am pleased!" and hugs me.

As PK cleanses you on the cellular level, you release old patterns. That includes cravings for foods, ways of thinking, family patterns. You move closer to your true essence, your Divine blueprint.

As I move on to breakfast, I feel contemplative and quiet, taking a few sips of my chai until I am more energized and able to listen to the conversations in the dining area. I sit in silence, eating my breakfast.

This morning the final phase of bodywork starts. As usual, the routine begins with the two-person body massage and oleation. But today it takes a new layer, as the special procedure done that day is meant to further prepare the body for the release. *Pishinchhali*, or as one ayurvedic technician from New Mexico refers to it, "pissinchili," has to be one of the messiest and most challenging of the various procedures I have ever experienced. Of course, there is a fair amount of oil involved. Along with the oil being poured onto your body, there is a rice ball wrapped in a cloth that Pravin uses to work the oil into my body. He is playing the Ganesha mantra and sings along as he is performing this vigorous procedure. I am smiling as he sings, amazed at his energy while he is doing this. And this is after a full week of up to ten clients each day receiving bodywork and shirodhara from him.

HOW IT WORKS

Pishinchhali

Pishinchhali is a body treatment done before *virechana*. Using a rice ball, lots of oil is intensely massaged into the body. This drives the oil into the body. It further calms the vata dosha. It assists in removing toxins in the joints as well as reducing muscle spasms. Due to its healing attributes, it can be administered apart from panchakarma as an independent body treatment over several consecutive days.

As is part of the process, I have to turn over at some point for the rest of the procedure to be completed on that side. Herein lies the challenge. Due to the messiness of the procedure, there is no sheet on the table so there is very little to hold on to or absorb the excess oil. It is just a wooden table with me covered in oil! How do I turn over without falling off the table? The answer is, "Ever so carefully!" And hold on to the sides of the table too. Pravin and Raju are there to catch me if need be but I feel a surge of "I can do this" energy and turn at just the right speed with minimal challenge! I chuckle and exclaim, "I did it!" In all the years of having the PK process, I have never fallen off. I would like to keep that simple trend going for me!

The pishinchhali procedure is one that can be done separate from the PK week. It is very good at calming vata down, which is easily aggravated, especially in hot, dry climates. It aids in eliminating toxins in the joints, and thus can improve mobility. It has helped to reduce muscle spasms as well. For the maximum benefit, this needs to be administered with some frequency over a short time period. That does not happen in this particular PK.

Then, there is pinda swedana, which is a procedure wherein a ball of rice and hot milk mixture is applied to the body in a cloth. This process aids in toning the muscles and ligaments. This is not as vigorous as the previous procedure, but I find both of them invigorating. I carefully make my way off the table to the bathroom and shower. It is indeed a messy procedure but I have enjoyed myself despite some of the challenges presented by the level of oil delivered on the table.

AYURVEDIC BODYWORK

Pinda Swedana

This procedure follows pishinchhali. A ball of rice, with herbs to calm vata dosha, is soaked and heated in milk. Wrapped in cloth, this rice ball is then rubbed over the entire body. The focus is on the muscles and joints, and the treatment takes about ten minutes.

Afterward, I return to my room. No other bodywork or basti will happen today, and no shirodhara. The idea is to rest the body and not to apply too much heat. It is almost lunchtime, but I hear that it is time for the consultation with Sunil. I am to take the herbs and tonics with me to be reviewed. I also bring with me notes and questions from the week.

In his office, Sunil asks about my appetite and my sleep, takes my blood pressure and pulse, and does a physical exam including palpation of the abdomen. My belly is nice and soft with no tender points. He gently pinches my skin on my arm and ankles, then notes, "You have taken in enough oil this week. I can see that when I pinch your skin!" He also notes that there is a slight sheen to the skin as well from all the oil ingestion and application.

Sunil then reviews the chart of each day, such as the elimination of the bowels over the week. This is very important as this is an indicator of how empty the colon is overall. If the colon is empty enough, the release that happens through the night is more complete. Sunil looks up at me with a smile, "You have had a good week with the preparation. You are on for *virechana!*"

This is one of the deciding factors, along with the level of oleation of the skin, as to whether virechana is an option that evening or not. And, of course, your mental state as to whether you feel strong enough to participate in the final phase.

As all goes well with the clinical assessment, I take the tracking form, which is given to me in order to have a written record of the events of the night. As Sunil hands it to me, he looks at me in a most sincere manner. "It is most important that you give me *all* the details of what I ask, which includes the time and volume of elimination, and the symptoms before and during the release. It is a guide to review how the physical release happened."

He adds, "The time at which the hand-rolled herbs are taken is critical for the release, as these herbs set the liver and gallbladder up for it."

The three main ingredients in the hand-rolled herbs are *cassia fistula* (Bahawa), *vitia vinifera* (Manuka) and *mallotus philipinaisis* (Kampillak).

The beauty of this process is that it is one of the safest ways to allow for a release to occur in the liver and gallbladder. It helps to minimize the challenges with gallstones, a concern for most people at some point in their lives. Sunil shares, "These herbs have been rolled during the time of the full moon by my mother, and there is much love and care in each of these herbs!"

What number of herbal pills to give? He has information from other PKs I have done. He looks up from the chart, "I think you can take four pills at 9 p.m. then four more at 9:30 p.m. You have taken that many before and done well!"

TENDER LOVING CARE

Fresh Rolled Herbs

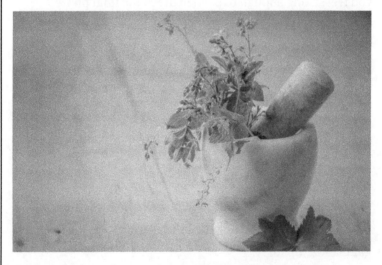

Bahawa, manuka, and kampillak are three fresh-rolled herbs that flush the liver.

Three principal herbs allow for the purging process to unfold with minimal effort. These hand-rolled herbs are *cassia fistula* (Bahawa), *vitia vinifera* (Manuka), and *mallotus philipinaisis* (Kampillak). They aid in the flushing of the liver at a volume that most people can tolerate. It's important to note that there is a natural stopping point for the purge once the accumulated toxins are gone.

I look at him and say, "I trust you to make the decision about this!"

He reminds me, saying, "Despite having done this process with thousands of people at this point, each time is different for each person. So when the beginning of the elimination phase is unknown, trust the wisdom of the body to start when it is best for you!"

What he is referring to is the fact that the herbs kick off a releasing process in the liver, but when it starts exactly in the middle of the night is unknown. It could be midnight or later. How often you will be up is also unknown. Just be prepared for what is possible and surrender to it is what is needed!

One last thing I ask is, "How much ghee or herbs tonight?"

Sunil reviews my chart of the week and says, "You have had enough ghee at this point. No more is needed, but if there is any cramping or nausea, do take some ginger tea and ½ teaspoon of ghee. And with your herbs, just take the ones for digestion as well as this loose herb, sukhasarek, to further aid in digestion." In this traditional ayurvedic herbal mixture, there is haritaki and senna with some mineral salts.

I pick up the hand-rolled herbs and the sheet to mark the events of the night. As I turn to leave, Sunil smiles broadly, saying, "May all go well with your virechana! I have prayed for all of you!"

I say, "I am most grateful to be here. It warms my heart to know that you have prayed for us."

He reminds me, saying, "You are the one giving yourself this gift. I thank you for making the journey and the commitment to have panchakarma done here in India!"

I am finished for the day, so I take time to visit with Sankara and Prema. We have spoken of sharing pictures of their daughter's wedding. Prema and I go into their room to view them. I see the flowers behind the wedding couple. Prema happily shares, saying, "The florist and crew came in at 3 a.m. the day of the wedding to make the frame of flowers. Beautiful white jasmine flowers with such an aroma. And they were only there for that part of the wedding, as other flowers and platforms were created for the rest of the ceremony."

Krishna and Radha

Krishna is a revered deity and avatar who is a flute carrier and is often depicted blue in his skin color. Once, a sister of Radha questioned her about the flute and why he carried his flute so close to his heart. "Why does Krishna carry his flute so close to the heart? Are you not worried?" Suddenly concerned, Radha said, "Who is number one in Krishna's heart?" She decided to ask him. Krishna said, "Of course, it is my flute!" Radha asked, "Why?" Krishna then said, "Because as the flute is empty, my heart is able to create whatever music it desires!"

Sunil told me this story when I arrived in Nagpur, one of many treasures awaiting me as I surrendered my body, mind, and soul to the experience.

———

Panchakarma is similar to the flute
that Krishna plays as it allows the body
(instrument/vehicle) to be emptied completely
so that it may be able to express itself, thus
connecting to the dharma that is meant to be.

———

The Anticipation

Only three of us will have virechana, so we come together to share a meal. This particular meal is meant to aid in creating enough bulk to further support the elimination process. I comment, "This is a great last meal before the big night!" The two others both laugh. Sankara points out, "The best is yet to come!" Both admit that they were a bit nervous about the night as it is ever so unpredictable.

I, too, find I am a little nervous, as their anxiety is infectious. A set of powdered herbs are delivered by a clinic staff person, and both Prema and I are to take them, but the written instructions are a little vague as to the time to ingest them. We end up calling Sunil to clarify. When we finally sort it out, I realize that I need to simply be in my own room, in my own space, so to be able to settle down. I normally do not become so distraught, but I realize I am more open and sensitive to those around me. And up to now, there has been no reason for concern.

I begin the evening ritual with the herbs and prepare for the night ahead. In addition to the herbs timed at 9 p.m. and 9:30 p.m., there is an electrolyte solution that needs to be prepared, as I need to hydrate when I wake up each time. Neetu has prepared simple, hot ginger tea, cut up ginger pieces to nibble on if I become nauseated, and a thermos of hot water. I prepare space on the desk in my room. I also remember to *not* take the prescribed ghee tonight.

I locate a basin to have handy, as it assists in helping measure how much I evacuate during the night. I know there are those who have refused to do so, but the way the toilet bowls are formed in India, it is hard to even guess how much is in the bowl. It is a straight shot down with the bowl being at a level not visible to my eyes. The basin sits nicely in the interior of the toilet. And dumping out the contents is as easy as tipping it.

As I prepare for bed, I feel calmer and ready for the last phase of the panchakarma treatment. Taking the first of the hand-rolled herbs, I notice the astringent, slightly bitter taste. The herbs are easy to chew and have a fresh quality. I have been ready to go to bed and sleep for about thirty minutes but there is one more set of herbs to take! I read a little and listen to some music as I wait for 9:30 p.m. to come around. I am most ready to turn off the light. I fall asleep easily after.

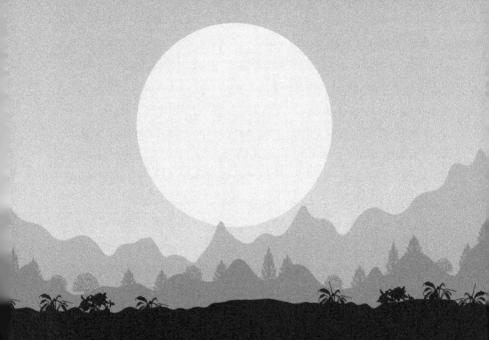

Chapter Eight

Open, Calm, Eager

CLARITY PRESENT
SENSES OPEN, RECEIVING
CALM AND RESONANT

DAY EIGHT

The virechana night ended up being kind to me. I had been able to fall asleep easily at 9:30 p.m. after taking the last of the four rolled herbs. I knew what to expect, which helps a little. Yet each time can be so different that there is a need to surrender to how the night unfolds. This ultimately aids in the process at the physiological level. By letting go mentally and emotionally, the body can then do what is needed with greater ease.

There is a sound inside me that alerts me to wake up. To me it sounds like a train is rumbling through my abdomen. It feels like it starts at the small intestine level under the rights side of my rib cage. I am suddenly pulled from deep sleep with this sensation of movement in my belly. This movement feels swift and "on a mission." There is no cramping. I sit up and recall where I am and what is happening tonight. I look at the clock and see it is 1:30 a.m. I then go to the "throne" of the night. The rumble has continued without cramping. I most easily evacuate my bowels. And continue and continue. The evacuation is swift and efficient, yet the volume is what always amazes me. I have had a basti every day this week and that led to having two or three, maybe four bowel movements daily. And though I eat three meals a day, the amount is probably closer to 1,500 calories per day with the meals being gluten-, dairy-, and soy-free except for the chapatis and the milk in the chai.

I realize I am "complete" for the moment. I attempt a visual measure of the volume of stool in the bowl. Noting the color of the stool, it is light brown and of a mushy quality. I do not remember the significance at that time of night, but I do write down the info and slide back to bed.

I sleep again easily. And the "train rumble" starts again around 4:30 a.m. No cramping is present. I repeat the process, and again a similar color presents, but the volume is quite diminished. I attempt to go back to bed but not long enough to go to sleep, as I am summoned again to seek the throne of the night. This pattern recurs for the next hour or so.

Eventually I fall into a deep sleep. I wake up near 7:30 a.m. I feel a little tired but considering the pattern of release and sleep the night before, I feel really good. I am feeling very light physically and emotionally. Few, if any, thoughts are roaming in my mind. Beginning my morning routine, I shower and prepare for the day. There are no herbs taken today. I am finished, without needing to take any more medicated ghee. I briefly meditate and offer prayers for the day and in gratitude for the ease of the night.

Today is a complete day of rest. No yoga is offered today. I hear a knock on my door, so I open it. It is Pravin, holding a cup of ginger tea for me. "How was your virechana?" he asks with a smile. I share with him that it went well enough and that I was able to have a good amount of undisturbed sleep. He then cautions me. "The toxins are still moving through and being released, so having this ginger tea and more throughout the day will help. It can reduce any nausea you may have."

He adds, "Rest now and throughout the day to conserve your energy, as the process is so complete in draining the body and brain."

I nod my head and say ,"I agree, as I know what has happened to me when I have not been respectful of the process in the past!"

In the past I have attempted to work some during this process, and returned full time to the activities that are required for work. It is a mighty challenge to do so. Most importantly, I have not honored myself and my needs in the process by taking the rest that is so necessary afterward. This time I have done what I needed to do to truly honor myself. Taking the time away from work and being present with the cleanse is a gift to me. It has deepened the experience that is possible with PK. I am better able to notice the gifts of clarity and awareness. The lightness of being is more apparent. My body is humming along. My being is more open.

I liken it to *savasana*. Being in the corpse pose after doing the asanas of yoga allows for the integration of all the benefits of the movements just performed. Rest is where the body and brain are able to rejuvenate. Similarly with our need for enough sleep daily!

Day of Rest

At about 8:30 a.m., I wander into the kitchen. This is a day of complete rest for the digestive system except for the simplest of preparations of rice. This part of the process is referred to *Samsarjana Krama*. As *agni* (digestive fire) is typically quite weak at this point after the virechana, this program offers steps to proceed with ease. This supports the gradual rebuilding of the agni. Refraining from certain foods and drinking ginger tea further aids the process. And most importantly, *I am not to eat unless I am hungry.* Drinking Recharge is an option as well. This is a healthier option than Gatorade. In India, I am given rehydration salts to put in a solution, as there is no Recharge here.

To start with, options for food include the rice-milk water known as *manda.* Drinking this milk water through the day until satisfied, but not beyond, is important. The next level of food is soft rice with spices known as *vilepi.* Small meals, again, are what is best at this point. The next level is soft rice and dal, referred to as *odan.* Then, the final offering is *kitchari,* which is rice and dal with spices and soft vegetables. It needs to be soft and creamy, which means adding more water to the recipe. To progress to less soft rice and cooked vegetables with minimal spicing, it is important to gauge how well you are digesting and how quickly your appetite returns. For me, my appetite typically returns by nightfall with a strong desire to eat.

With PK, you can find a new equilibrium that stays in your being. Old habits that are not supportive of you are easy to drop. New choices are now possible.

Neetu is present, preparing breakfast. Smiling, she asks, "How was your night?"

I reply, "Easier than I anticipated! I actually slept most of the night except at the 1:30 a.m. and 4:30 a.m. releases!"

She hands me rice water to sip on. "This is the first stage to slowly reintroduce food." She then shows me the next food items I am to ingest. It is just rice that has been cooked to a soft mush. I do notice that I am not very hungry, but welcome the rice water as I am thirsty!

Neetu points to the pot on the burner. I am able to have *kitchari* once my appetite returns during the day, but no other foods for now.

Years earlier, I learned from Sunil and Gerhardt Horstman, the main ayurvedic technician in the US for the program in Albuquerque, of the diet for transitioning to other foods. Each phase has a specific type of rice recipe for the transition. My digestion afterward is usually quite strong. This is true this time as well.

I feel tired, but nourished with the rice options I am offered. And I already feel the desire for more substantive food. I return to my room to rest and to wait to hear from Sunil Joshi for my exit interview.

I am feeling a tenderness and fragility, both emotionally and physically. I find that resting with my eyes covered is my favorite pose of the day. I take a walk but find that it only fatigues me more.

Mukul comes to my room to inform me that Sunil is ready to see me. He smiles and asks, "How are you doing?"

I smile and give him a hug, saying, "I am good but tired. I know that I need to rest a lot today!"

He replies, "Good of you to say that, as you work hard and you need your rest for now." I follow him downstairs and sit in the waiting area.

The waiting area has two brown love seats and a low glass-topped table. There are booklets about the local temple along with the family's guru. The lighting is low, with the dark-brown curtain drawn. It feels cool and calm. Ganesha sits in the corner with flowers to honor his presence in the clinic. The small herbal pharmacy on site is bustling with activity as staff members prepare the final herbs I will take home with me. I listen to the Ganesha CD playing in the background. It is one of my favorite mantras, and I note the track is on the CD I purchased a few days earlier. I am feeling excited to hear from Sunil as to how the night unfolded for me. His clinical acumen shines here as this is where he sees the biggest changes in people.

How Did I Do?

Mukul summons me to Sunil's office, where Sunil greets me with a big smile. He asks, "How was your virechana?"

I smile as well and state, "It was incredibly gentle this time for me, and I even slept a fair amount!"

He exclaims, "Good! Let's see how you did!" I hand him the sheet with all the intimate details of the night. He looks at the chart and then shares, "Again, thank you for coming so far to do PK! You did great!"

He analyzes the external indicators to see how well the release went. I have noted these indicators on the data sheet through the night: What part of the night were you up for the bowels to release? How often were you up? What were your symptoms at the time of release? Did you feel discomfort? gurgling? cramping? headache? Did you notice any stones in the stool content? Yes...you are asked to view the content of each stool and to measure to the best of your ability by a visual guess at the quantity in the basin you are given to place in the toilet!

Sunil begins to examine my pulses on both wrists with three fingers, lifting each one gently as he palpates at different levels. He makes some notes in the chart.

As Sunil peruses the chart, my eyes wander around the office. He is seated behind a large brown office desk with a glass top. There is medical information in the form of articles posted there, as well as pictures of the colon with disease present. There is also a stethoscope. To his left sits a large vintage telephone that has a broken clock. There is a shrine in the back corner with a picture of Sri Ramakrishna and Mataji. Bhagawan's picture is there as well. The deity present is Hanuman. The ghee lamp burns in honor of these guides. The reverence for these holy men and women in Sunil's life is evident. It warms my heart to be present in this room, especially after the night I just experienced. I feel very open and vulnerable.

After Sunil finishes his review of my chart, he looks up. "Please come to the exam table," he says, and I move from my chair to the table. He palpates my abdomen and notes, "It feels soft and empty!"

I agree and share, "There is no tenderness where you are palpating."

He takes out the blood pressure cuff from the drawer next to the table. He places the cuff on my right arm. As he pumps it up, I notice some sadness coming up for me. As he checks the numbers, he shares that my blood pressure is normal for me.

I sit up and return to my seat. As Sunil launches into an explanation of what he sees, he states, "You have shifted very nicely. Your vata and pitta dosha have come down nicely. And most importantly, your kapha dosha has finally started to increase. This is most important as this dosha is one of cohesion and is part of your *prakruti*," i.e. it is closer to the constitution at the time of my birth. As he explains what this means, I again notice how tender I feel. And begin to cry.

Sunil looks at me gently and says, "You have opened up a lot during this week. You are coming from the heart even more, and with the kapha dosha coming forth, this will aid in the resilience in your being. Be gentle with yourself!"

I nod through my tears, "I agree with you about my heart opening, and am grateful for my resilience coming through more!"

He recalls that I am traveling on from Nagpur to the southern Himalayas. He strongly recommends that I be careful with my dietary choices as I move north and away from the ayurvedic cooking that has been so readily available here. Key for me to remember: minimal spicing, minimal yogurt unless it is fresh, as it could include buttermilk. In the past, I have basically eaten rice, cooked vegetables, and roti along with bottled water, chai, and ginger tea. Making these choices has allowed me to enjoy having no digestive problems during my trips to India. I have added fresh yogurt in the morning, but only if it is available.

Sunil reviews my herbs for digestion and for support for daily stress. The digestive herbs have been most effective for me. I have not needed any Western medications and experience very strong digestion of the foods I choose to eat. I find this key to my daily lifestyle. One's ability to have healthy digestion of food in the body is most important for overall health and well being. I have greater clarity in my thinking. I am not sluggish or tired after meals, mentally or physically. There is no bloating and gas. I have not needed any Western medications for digestive problems or acid reflux. The Western medications only suppress symptoms; they do not get to the root of the issue. With ayurvedic herbs, I am supported in a manner that is holistic and balancing for me.

Another herb that has been most helpful is an adaptogen. Sunil has added one specific one, ashwagandha, to my herbal regimen. This is a particular herb that has many amazing qualities for supporting immunity and mental well-being. For me, ashwagandha has been a mainstay for me in the months after PK. This is an adaptogen that is quite calming and assists the adrenals if there is any adrenal fatigue present. At times, more than one adaptogen can be given.

FOOD AS MEDICINE

Rasayana Jam

This mixture of over fifty herbs has been has been slow cooked and is used as a jam to add to tea or toast. Taken one or two times a day, it bolsters the rejuvenation that can occur after PK and helps to maintain a sense of strength and well-being.

Additionally, there has been enough of a shift in my doshas that a *rasayana* jam is now a part of my herb regimen. This particular herbal combination is part of the maintenance program that rejuvenates after panchakarma. It keeps the person active mentally and physically—and more youthful.

They prescribed me with an oil made from a combination of coconut and sesame, with herbs that have been cooked with oil. I will continue the daily oleation that I have practiced here at the clinic. I know I can purchase this oil at the Albuquerque center, but just the same, I purchased three months' worth of herbs. It costs far less here. Plus, the herbs are monitored for any heavy metals and other possible contaminants.

As I leave, I give Sunil a hug. I feel sad as I know that the care, along with the quality of food I have received, will not be soon replicated for me. I am about to embark on another three weeks in India, a journey into the unknown. I plan to go to a Divine Feminine Shakti retreat to the Himalayas for ten days. I feel very open and aware in this moment. I am excited about what else may unfold in this journey. I feel a sense of anticipation. I also know that I have support from the clinic if need be during my stay in India. That offers comfort to me, as I will be traveling alone.

CRIMES AGAINST WISDOM

No Leftovers

No leftovers are recommended, as the food is considered old and believed to have little life force or prana and is thus not able to nourish the body. The fresher the food, the more alive it is and the better; the closer to the source you are, the more this is so; homemade is the best, having your meal prepared by those who love you.

I return to my room and know that I am to visit with my newly made friends for one last time. We are all leaving in the next two days. I leave to go north to Delhi and they return home to Chennai. I am eager to finish some of the stories we had begun to share, but also to hear how their cleanses went.

I find them in the kitchen having ginger tea, but see they are hopeful to have some chai. They are in conversation with Neetu, who has returned to start the evening meal. Neetu shakes her head, "No chai until tomorrow, as it is too late in the day for chai and the milk is too heavy for all of you after virechana!" But she informs us, "There is to be rice, dal, and chapatis for dinner." This is a sign that each of us already has a robust *agni*, as all of us loudly voice our hunger pangs.

I laugh as I hear this about the chai (but am happy to hear about being able to have regular food). We are funny as humans. We can be eager to push the envelope, but today is one day to have true respect for the boundary that is in place for us.

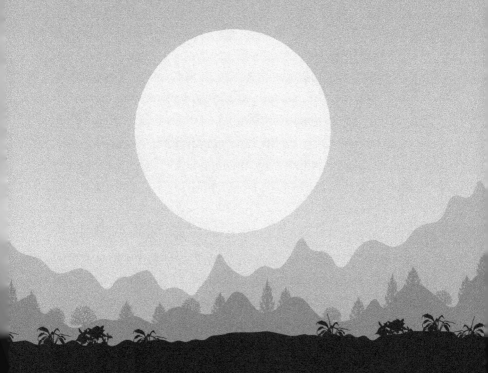

Chapter Nine

Life Ever After

REJUVENATED
REFRESHED, RESET, AND RENEWED
BEAUTY IN AND OUT

Now that the week and the significant night are over, what is next? First and foremost, it is most important to be as gentle with yourself as possible. This includes being cautious in returning to old habits that were there before the cleanse. I know that my digestion is quite sensitive afterwards. Making wise choices early on can ease the transition back to daily life back home.

Before I leave Nagpur, I meet with Sunil, who emphasizes this. I hear it from Pravin as soon as he sees me in the morning after virechana. Pacing myself can be a challenge, and yet, after a cleanse of this depth, it is most necessary.

The cleanse is profound for me in so many ways. With each subsequent one, I am more aware, more present, and find the process to be even gentler on my body. And as more of my body is balanced, my mental and emotional layers are more balanced. My body has been through a deep and profound flush that goes to the cellular level. The doshas and the dhatus have become anew. Rejuvenation is now possible. The resulting impact on my emotions is that I experience more equanimity and am perturbed less. My mind is thus more able to access the quiet within and reach the higher self. This lends to a sense of wholeness and clarity. I feel more at ease with myself. Each day, I look forward to how my day unfolds.

In the days after this PK, I feel quite luminous. Literally, I feel this light emanating from me and from my eyes. I hear from others who notice the same. I hold a lightness of being and a lightheartedness that I truly enjoy. My heart feels wide open, and as I walk outside of the clinic, I easily smile at the families and individuals walking by. I have no agenda but to walk down the street. I enjoy being so present and alive. I swear that I think I can hear my cells humming along with me.

Epilogue

Returning to Life

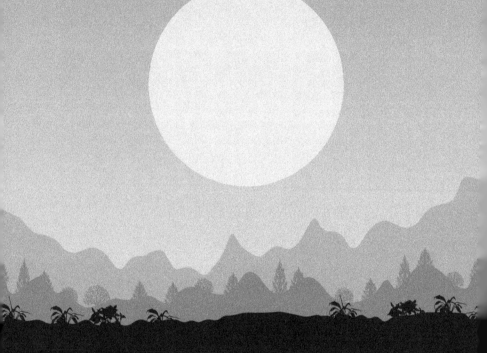

WISDOM SAYS THAT I AM NOTHING.
LOVE SAYS THAT I AM EVERYTHING.
INSTEAD OF SEARCHING FOR WHAT YOU DO NOT HAVE,
FIND OUT WHAT IT IS YOU NEVER LOST.
IF YOU CHANGE YOURSELF,
YOU WILL FIND THAT NO OTHER CHANGE IS NEEDED.

—SRI NISARGADATTA MAHARAJ

On this journey, I returned to my soul. But I also returned to a new life. Longstanding patterns were no longer present, and I know this profoundly because in the year that came after, I made many changes, significant and subtle, in the structure of my life, be it the pattern of pleasing others at the expense of myself or the pattern of creeping in fear of failure, moving beyond my current paradigm into this new realm of soul expression. I have found that which was never lost, simply covered up, shielded by these patterns, layers present most of my lifetime.

I knew this, even in those first days after the PK. I knew that returning to the structure of my life in the United States after such a profound change could be unsettling, to say the least. I had found that before. And I think it's particularly true of returning to the Western world. After India, returning to my own culture had a very different twist. The life I had been living no longer resonated for me. I knew deep in my heart and soul that things needed to change. I needed to shift in a profound way—at all levels of my being. And it began with living and being present in a graceful, honest way with my soul.

In those first few days, I made a vow to remember to attune to the rhythm of my days. Upon my return, I would adjust to the time change and make a point of getting up in the morning with enough time to perform simple asanas and a meditation along with pranayama. I have implemented this routine and maintained it. I find that it creates a foundation for my day. I know that this is as important as my physical hygiene. This hygienic routine of asanas and meditation supports my mental and emotional hygiene. And in creating this ritual, I plant the seeds for the day and the next day, for my ability to weather what is tossed at me on a day to day basis, and to do so with a certain amount of grace.

My choices in diet and food preparation are important changes to consider. This is foundational in order for the effects of PK to last and to reduce the amount of ama that can accumulate in the body. Simple changes can have a beneficial impact. Eating freshly prepared foods daily, including cooked/ steamed vegetables, preferably at home, is an excellent beginning. Adding a healthy oil such as olive oil into the cooking or as a light condiment brings in the necessary fats our body and brain need. Eating in a pleasant, quieter environment allows for the reduction of sensory stimulation and easier digestion. Avoiding refined foods or fast foods for a variety of reasons is a good thing to consider; one reason is that these foods are very hard for the body to digest. Another is that they create more ama, which settles into the different tissue layers in the body leading to chronic disease. Remember that this cleanse has helped to remove the ama from the seven *dhatus/* layers in the body, so limiting fast or processed food would be a gift for your physical body. Often the cravings of these foods can be gone after panchakarma.

For me, limiting fried foods of any kind further supports the pitta dosha and helps to keep it in balance. Fasting every two weeks for a half day to a whole day, with broth or vegetables, is a practice I now do to keep the *agni* (fire) stronger, which aids in digestion. This type of fasting is much easier for me than some other fasting options like a water fast.

Other ways to support changes in this new phase of life include seeing where else there are toxic elements in the life one is returning to. Remember the questions I asked early on? They have new meaning after PK as you have changed internally so much. Here is the list again for you to consider: How toxic are the people with whom I choose to spend time? How toxic is the environment where I live or work? How toxic are my thoughts? How toxic is the music to which I listen? How many hours of the news cycle do I watch, only to become more distressed mentally and emotionally? Do I sit with my family for a meal without the television? Am I so absorbed with the electronics in my life that I have neglected the ones with whom I live and share a dwelling?

Why bother with all of these details?

As human beings, we are made of the same elements as nature. Ayurveda has shown us that by understanding how these elements of nature dance, we have clear approaches to help us regain the balance and health that is intrinsic in the wisdom of the body. For each of us, given our unique perspective and depending on what doshas we are given, this process acts a roadmap for us as individuals to be able to make choices that are best for *us*! The end goal with this selectivity and thoughtfulness is an incredible level of *preventative* self-healthcare unknown to the Western world before the past twenty years or so. And often, this starts with the diet/food choices that are most supportive for you and your specific dosha.

All these changes of diet can happen without panchakarma. Yet, panchakarma jump-starts the process, removing patterns at the cellular level. This helps with aspects of the rejuvenation process that can be most beneficial.

In addition, these ayurvedic supportive interventions allow for reduction in pain and suffering from chronic illnesses, and thus a greater level of health and quality of life. As there is more and more evidence that our modern lifestyle leads to greater levels of chronic disease, Panchakarma and an ayurvedic lifestyle shift can be a resource for those suffering from these diseases. This would be a move toward wellness.

The steps of self-care are present in Ayurveda. Ayurveda makes possible an increased awareness of health and the knowledge of how to care for the gift of our human body. Improved health is possible, if not rejuvenation. May your choices support you to have a happy, healthy, blissful life.

When I began this journey with PK, I had no idea about the depth of the changes that are possible. I needed to have four of them, along with a health scare, before I noticed patterns being released, including old emotional patterns with my family that no longer served me. In addition, my clarity of thinking has consistently improved. My health overall remains good.

The journey that I have been on has only become better and better with a sense of being present in my life. I am more creative and happier with decisions I have made. Joy is present in my heart, which sings to the dawn of each new day. I treasure the blessings I have in my life even more.

Om Namah Shivaya.

Appendix A

Blank Ritual Journal

ROUTINES

	M	T	W	T	F	S	S
_____	○	○	○	○	○	○	○
_____	○	○	○	○	○	○	○
_____	○	○	○	○	○	○	○
_____	○	○	○	○	○	○	○
_____	○	○	○	○	○	○	○
_____	○	○	○	○	○	○	○
_____	○	○	○	○	○	○	○
_____	○	○	○	○	○	○	○
_____	○	○	○	○	○	○	○
_____	○	○	○	○	○	○	○
_____	○	○	○	○	○	○	○
_____	○	○	○	○	○	○	○
_____	○	○	○	○	○	○	○
_____	○	○	○	○	○	○	○
_____	○	○	○	○	○	○	○
_____	○	○	○	○	○	○	○
_____	○	○	○	○	○	○	○

OIL

	M	T	W	T	F	S	S
_____	○	○	○	○	○	○	○
_____	○	○	○	○	○	○	○
_____	○	○	○	○	○	○	○
_____	○	○	○	○	○	○	○
_____	○	○	○	○	○	○	○
_____	○	○	○	○	○	○	○
_____	○	○	○	○	○	○	○
_____	○	○	○	○	○	○	○
_____	○	○	○	○	○	○	○
_____	○	○	○	○	○	○	○
_____	○	○	○	○	○	○	○
_____	○	○	○	○	○	○	○
_____	○	○	○	○	○	○	○
_____	○	○	○	○	○	○	○
_____	○	○	○	○	○	○	○
_____	○	○	○	○	○	○	○
_____	○	○	○	○	○	○	○

CLEANSES

	M	T	W	T	F	S	S
_____	○	○	○	○	○	○	○
_____	○	○	○	○	○	○	○
_____	○	○	○	○	○	○	○
_____	○	○	○	○	○	○	○
_____	○	○	○	○	○	○	○
_____	○	○	○	○	○	○	○
_____	○	○	○	○	○	○	○
_____	○	○	○	○	○	○	○
_____	○	○	○	○	○	○	○
_____	○	○	○	○	○	○	○
_____	○	○	○	○	○	○	○
_____	○	○	○	○	○	○	○
_____	○	○	○	○	○	○	○
_____	○	○	○	○	○	○	○
_____	○	○	○	○	○	○	○
_____	○	○	○	○	○	○	○

FOOD AS MEDICINE

	M	T	W	T	F	S	S
_____	○	○	○	○	○	○	○
_____	○	○	○	○	○	○	○
_____	○	○	○	○	○	○	○
_____	○	○	○	○	○	○	○
_____	○	○	○	○	○	○	○
_____	○	○	○	○	○	○	○
_____	○	○	○	○	○	○	○
_____	○	○	○	○	○	○	○
_____	○	○	○	○	○	○	○
_____	○	○	○	○	○	○	○
_____	○	○	○	○	○	○	○
_____	○	○	○	○	○	○	○
_____	○	○	○	○	○	○	○
_____	○	○	○	○	○	○	○
_____	○	○	○	○	○	○	○
_____	○	○	○	○	○	○	○
_____	○	○	○	○	○	○	○

MOVEMENT

	M	T	W	T	F	S	S
_____	○	○	○	○	○	○	○
_____	○	○	○	○	○	○	○
_____	○	○	○	○	○	○	○
_____	○	○	○	○	○	○	○
_____	○	○	○	○	○	○	○
_____	○	○	○	○	○	○	○
_____	○	○	○	○	○	○	○
_____	○	○	○	○	○	○	○
_____	○	○	○	○	○	○	○
_____	○	○	○	○	○	○	○
_____	○	○	○	○	○	○	○
_____	○	○	○	○	○	○	○
_____	○	○	○	○	○	○	○
_____	○	○	○	○	○	○	○
_____	○	○	○	○	○	○	○
_____	○	○	○	○	○	○	○
_____	○	○	○	○	○	○	○

MEDITATION

	M	T	W	T	F	S	S
_____	○	○	○	○	○	○	○
_____	○	○	○	○	○	○	○
_____	○	○	○	○	○	○	○
_____	○	○	○	○	○	○	○
_____	○	○	○	○	○	○	○
_____	○	○	○	○	○	○	○
_____	○	○	○	○	○	○	○
_____	○	○	○	○	○	○	○
_____	○	○	○	○	○	○	○
_____	○	○	○	○	○	○	○
_____	○	○	○	○	○	○	○
_____	○	○	○	○	○	○	○
_____	○	○	○	○	○	○	○
_____	○	○	○	○	○	○	○
_____	○	○	○	○	○	○	○
_____	○	○	○	○	○	○	○
_____	○	○	○	○	○	○	○

Appendix A

Glossary

Abhyanga: Daily oil massage to increase circulation, decrease dryness and reduce *vata* aggravation.

Abhyantar Snehana: Internal oleation. Part of *Purvakarma* (the preparatory procedures of *Panchakarma),* it is specifically designed to liquefy and dislodge *ama* from the *dhatus.*

Agni: The element and universal organizing principle of conversion, light, and heat.

Agni Swedana: A procedure used to promote sweating and dilation of channels through heating the body.

Ahara: The Ayurvedic knowledge of proper diet. One of the three pillars of Ayurveda.

Akash: The element and universal organizing principle of space.

Alochak Pitta: The metabolic function associated with the eye.

Ama: The toxic residue of undigested food that is the source of illness in the body.

Anuloman: The aspect of gastrointestinal vitality concerned with proper elimination.

Anztwasan Basti: An oil *basti* which is meant to be retained in the colon for a long period of time.

Apana Vayu: The *sub-dosha* of *vata* which governs the elimination of waste.

Asanas: Hatha yoga postures designed to refine physiological functioning.

Asatmya-Indriyartha-Sarnyog: The improper uses of the senses.

Asthi: The *dhatu* or bodily tissue of bone.

Atma: The universal intelligence of nature. Also known as *param atma.*

Aushadhi: The Ayurvedic management of disease. One of the three pillars of Ayurveda.

Avapidana Nasya: Herbal mixtures crushed and squeezed into the nostrils.

Ayurveda: The science of life, the oldest health-care science known to man.

Bahya Snehana: External oleation used during *Purvakarma* (the preparatory procedures of *Panchakarrna),* specifically designed to liquefy and dislodge *arna* from the *dhatus.*

Bashpa Swedana: Steam bath. Part of the preparatory procedures of *Panchakarrna* specifically used to dilate the *shrotas* or channels of the body to facilitate the removal of *arna.*

Basti: Therapeutic purification and rejuvenation of the colon. One of the five main procedures of *Panchakarrna.*

Bheda: The sixth stage of disease manifestation characterized by complications.

Bhrajak Pitta: The metabolic function associated with the skin.

Bhutas: The five elements.

Bruhan Nasya: Medicated oil introduced into the nostrils to nourish both the senses and the brain.

Chandan Bala Oil: Medicated oil used in *bahya snehana* to pacify *pitta dosha.*

Charaka: The original commentator on Ayurveda, considered to be the father of Ayurveda.

Charaka Samhita: The first and most authoritative commentary on Ayurveda.

Dal: Split yellow mung lentil soup.

Deepan: The aspect of gastrointestinal vitality concerned with promoting strong digestive fire.

Dharma: Lifes purpose.

Dhatu Agni: The metabolic function associated with each of the seven *dhatus.*

Dhatus: The seven retainable substances or structures of the body. Bodily tissues.

Dhi: Intellect. The aspect of *sattva* that imparts the ability to conceive and imagine.

Dhruti: The positive aspect of *rajas* that imparts the ability to implement creative thought.

Dinacharya: Daily behavioral guidelines for maintaining ideal health.

Dusha: The functional intelligence within the human body responsible for all physiological and psychological processes.

Dusha Gati: The twice daily movement that each *dusha* follows from the hollow structures of the gastrointestinal tract to the thicker structures of the *dhatus* and back again. Also the movement of the *doshas* from their seats in the GI tract to their nearest orifice.

Drava Swedana: The use of hot baths to promote sweating.

Dwandaj: A condition where two *doshas* have an equally dominant influence in a person's *prakruti* or constitutional make-up.

Gandush: Gargling with a warm saline solution.

Gati: Mobility.

Ghee: Clarified butter.

Gunas: The three phases of activity in creation as well as the three qualities of the mind.

Indriyas: The five senses. One of the four components of Ayu.

Jaggery: Dried, unprocessed sugarcane juice.

Jala: The element and universal organizing principle of liquidity and cohesion. Also known as the water element.

Jathara Agni: The digestive fire, located in the gastrointestinal tract.

jiva Atma: The individual soul. One of the four components of Ayu.

Kai Basti: A *basti* that is administered at a specific time for maximum effect.

Kapha: The *dosha* or functional intelligence within the body governing cohesion, liquidity and growth.

Kapikachhu: An herb used to improve the function of *shukra dhatu.*

Karma: An action or procedure used in *Panchakarma* therapy.

Karma Basti: A month-long *basti* regimen administered to treat *vata-related* disorders.

Katti Basti: An external, localized application of medicated oil used in the region of the back.

Kaya Kalpa: Ancient rejuvenation procedure.

Kichari: A mixture of *basmati* rice and split yellow mung *dal* used to cleanse and balance the *doshas* during *Panchakarrna* therapy.

Ksheer Basti: A medicated milk decoction administered through the rectum which nourishes all the *dhattis* of the body.

Lekhana Basti: A strong, penetrating, cleansing *basti,* used specifically to reduce *kapha dosha* and *rneda dhatu.*

Lichen planus syndrome: A skin disease.

Mahabhutas: The universal organizing principles which structure and govern all physical phenomena.

Mahanarayana Oil: A medicated oil used in *bahya snehana* (the external oleation procedures of *Purvakarma)* specifically to pacify *kapha dosha.*

Majja: The *dhatu* or bodily tissue of bone marrow. Also, the term used to describe the bone marrow fat used on occasion in *abyantar snehana* (internal oleation).

Mala: The natural metabolic by-products which are always eliminated from the body.

Mamsa: The *dhatu* or bodily tissue of muscle.

Manas: The mind. One of the four components of *Ayu.*

Manda: Rice water. The first meal eaten after *Panchakarma.*

Manna: Sensitive points which represent a greater concentration of the body's vital force in that area.

Marsha Nasya: Repeated introduction of medicated oil into the nostrils used to clean, lubricate and strengthen the mucous membranes.

Matra Basti: A small self-administered oil *basti* that can be used at any time of the day, most commonly used to reduce the vata-aggravating effects of travel, exercise and stress.

Meda: The *dhatu* or bodily tissue of fat (adipose tissue).

Nadis: Very fine *shrotas* or channels of the body.

Nadi Swedana: Localized, penetrating steam administered specifically to the joints and spinal area during *Purvakarma.*

NaJya: The therapeutic cleansing of the head and neck region. One of the five purificatory procedures of *Panchakarma.*

Netra Basti: An external, localized application of medicated *ghee* around the eyes used to nourish the eyes, reduce eye strain and improve vision.

Netra Tarpana: Same as *Netra Basti.*

Nirooha Basti: A large, herbalized decoction administered into the colon to remove toxins and wastes from the body.

Ojakshaya: Depletion of *ojas.*

Ojas: the most refined product of *dhatu* metabolism which controls the body's immune function.

Pachak Pitta: The metabolic function occurring in the small intestine.

Pachan: The aspect of gastrointestinal vitality concerned with improving digestion and metabolism.

Pakwashaya Gata Basti: Basti administered through the rectum. The main type of *basti* used in *Panchakarma.*

Panchakarma: The five major purificatory procedures and adjunct therapies for purifying and rejuvenating the body.

Panchamahabhuta: The theory of the five elements.

Panchendriya Vardhan Oil: Oil used in *nasya* to nourish sensory functioning.

Param Atma: The universal intelligence of nature.

Parinam: The negative effects of the seasons on the body. The third major cause of disease after *pragya aparadha* and *astmya-indriyartha-samyog.*

Paryushit: Food that no longer contains vital force or *prana Paschatkarma:* The post-procedures of *Panchakarrna* therapy.

Peya: Rice soup. The second meal eaten after the main procedures of *Panchakarma* have been administered.

Pinda Swedana: A fomentation procedure performed with a bolus of rice and a hot milk decoction to tonify the muscles and improve the circulation.

Pishinchhali: A vigorous herbal massage using a bolus of rice and a large amount of oil to improve the mobility of muscles and ligaments.

Pitta: The *dosha* or functional intelligence within the body governing all metabolic processes.

Pragya aparadha: The mistake of the intellect. Considered by Ayurveda to be the foremost cause of disease.

Prakopa: The second stage of disease manifestation characterized by provocation or aggravation of *ama* at its site of origin (in the G-I tract).

Prakruti: The inherent balance of *doshas* that is most beneficial to one's life. The constitution we are born with.

Prana: life-force or vital force.

Prana Vayu: The *sub-dosha* of *Vata* which governs sensory functions and the intake of *prana,* water and food.

Pranayama: An alternate nostril breathing exercise which increases the intake of *prana.* One of the three exercises of *vyayama.*

Prapaka Metabolism: The three transient phases of digestion that take place in the gastrointestinal tract.

Prasara: The third stage of disease manifestation characterized by the migration of *ama* from its site of origin (in the G-I tract).

Prati Marsha Nasya: Repeated application of medicated oil to the nostrils with the tip of the little finger to soothe dry mucous membranes and to protect against airborne allergens.

Prithvi: The element and universal organizing principle of form and structure. Also commonly known as the earth element.

Purvakarma: The set of procedures used to prepare a person for the main purificatory procedures of *Panchakarma*.

Rajas: The active phase of the mind. It imparts motivation and initiative to the mind. Also one of the three *gunas* or phases of activity in creation.

Rajasic: Pertaining to the qualities of *rajas*.

Rakta: The *dhatu* or bodily tissue of blood.

Raktarnokshana: Therapeutic withdrawal of blood. One of the five major purificatory procedures of *Panchakarrna*.

Ranjak Pitta: The metabolic function associated with the liver.

Rasa: The *dhatu* or bodily tissue of plasma or nutrient fluid. Also refers to the three categories of taste.

Rasayana: One of the branches of Ayurvedic science having to do with rejuvenation.

Rasayana Basti: A type of *basti* which has a rejuvenative influence on all the *dhatus*.

Rutucharya: The diet and lifestyle regimen prescribed by *vihara* to take into account the impact of each of the seasons on the body.

Sadhak Pitta: The metabolic function which controls the neuropeptides in the brain as well as mental processes.

Saindhava: Black salt.

Samana Vay: The *sub-dosha* of *vata* which governs the metabolism and distribution of nutrients in the body.

Samsarajana krama: The graded administration of diet. One of the post-procedures of *Panchakarma* concerned with strengthening the debilitated digestive fire.

Sanchaya: The first stage of disease manifestation characterized by the accumulation of *arna* in the gastrointestinal tract.

Sattva: The creative phase of the mind. The quality that imparts curiosity, inspiration and creativity to the mind. One of the three *gunas* or phases of activity in creation.

Sattvic: Pertaining to the qualities of *sattva*.

Shamana Basti: A therapeutic administration of medicated oil or decoction through the rectum to reduce irritation in the colon.

Sharnana Chikitsa: One of the two primary methods of disease management whose purpose is only to palliate the symptoms of disease.

Sharnana Nasya: A therapeutic administration of herbalized oil into the nostrils to soothe the sinus zone.

Sharira: The human body. One of the four components of *Ayu.*

Shat Kriya Kai: The six stages of disease manifestation.

Shiro Basti: Medicated oil administered to head which improves *prana* and sensory functioning.

Shirodhara: One of the adjunct procedures of *Purvakarrna* designed to calm the mind and pacify *vata* in the central nervous system.

Shirovirechana: Therapeutic cleansing of head and neck region. Also called *Nasya,* it is one of the five main purificatory procedures of *Panchakarma.*

Shodhana Basti: A therapeutic administration of medicated decoctions to cleanse the colon of toxic substances and waste products.

Shodhana Chikitsa: One of the two primary methods of disease management whose focus is to eliminate the source of disease.

Shodhana Nasya: A therapeutic administration of medicated oil into the nostrils to eliminate toxins from the paranasal sinus zone.

Shrotas: The gross and subtle channels of the body.

Shukra: The male and female reproductive tissue
of the body.

Smriti: Memory. More specifically, the positive aspect of
tamas that imparts the ability to remember those things
that are beneficial for our lives.

Sthana Samshraya: The fourth stage of disease
manifestation characterized by augmentation of the
disease process.

Surya Namaskar: Sun salutation in *Hatha Yoga asanas.*

Sushruta: One of the main commentators of Ayurvedic
science after *Charaka,* whose focus was surgical
procedures and purification of the blood.

Sushruta Samhita: Sushruta commentary on Ayurveda.

Swedana: One of the two main *Purvakarmas* (preparatory
procedures of *Panchakarma)* whose purpose is to
dilate the channels of the body so that the *doshas* can
easily transport the dislodged *ama* back to the GI tract
for elimination.

Tai/a: Oil.

Tamas: The phase in the mind that brings activity to an end.
It imparts dullness and inertia to the mind and causes a
loss of knowingness. One of the three *gunas* or phase of
activity in creation.

Tamasic: Pertaining to the quality of *tamas.*

Tapa Swedana: The application of dry heat to the body to reduce inflammation and congestion in the joints.

Tikta Ghrita: Medicated *ghee* with a predominantly bitter taste used in *abyantar snehana* (internal oleation) to remove *arna* from the *dhatus*.

Ti! Oil: Sesame oil.

Triphala: A laxative, combination of three fruits.

Udana Vayu: One of the *sub-doshas* of *vayu* which governs strength, speech and the elimination of carbon dioxide.

Udvartana: A type of therapeutic massage using powder instead of oil to reduce *rneda dhatu* and excess *kapha*.

Upanaha Swedana: A therapeutic application of warm, medicated poultices used to treat arthritis.

Uro Basti: Medicated oils that are retained on the chest and heart area to reduce congestion.

Utkleshana Basti: Therapeutic administration of medicated decoctions through the rectum to promote secretions in the colon which liquefy and expel *arna* and waste material.

Vagabhata: A major commentator on Ayurvedic science after *Charaka* and *Sushruta*.

Vaidya: An Ayurvedic physician.

Vaisharnya: The proportionate influence of the *doshas* that allows us to perceive the predominance of one over the others.

Vajirarana Basti: A *basti* which promotes vigor and vitality. Also used to enhance fertility.

Vamana: Therapeutic vomiting or emesis. One of the five main purificatory procedures of *Panchakarma*.

Vasa: An oleated substance composed of animal fat used in *abhyantar snehana* (internal oleation).

Vata: The *dosha* or functional intelligence in the body that governs movement, transportation and the drying and separating functions.

Vata Shamak Oil: The medicated oil used in *bahya snehana* (one of the main procedures of *Purvakarma)* to pacify *vata*.

Vayu: The element and universal organizing principle of movement. Also commonly known as the air or wind element.

Veda: The knowledge of the totality of life.

Vihara: The Ayurvedic knowledge of proper lifestyle. One of the three pillars of Ayurveda.

Vikruti: The imbalance in the *doshas* that obscures one's *prakrttti* or ideal constitutional balance.

Vilepi: Thick soup of soft cooked rice usually eaten on the second day after *Panchakarma.*

Vipaka: The post-absorptive phase of digestion.

Virechana: Therapeutic purgation. One of the five main purificatory procedures of *Panchakarma.*

Vranagata Basti: Medicated liquids used to irrigate and heal abscesses or wounds.

Vyakta: The fifth stage of disease manifestation characterized by the manifestation of a clear set of symptoms.

Vyana Vayu: One of the *sub-doshas* of *Vata* which governs the cardiovascular system.

Vyayama: Three exercises prescribed by *vihara* which give energy rather than expend energy: *hatha yoga* postures, *pranayama* and sun salutation.

Yog Basti: An eight-day oil *basti* regimen specifically designed to calm *vata* and nourish the colon.

Yusha: Dal (yellow mung lentil soup) eaten on the second day after *Panchakarma.*

Appendix B

Reasons to Consider PK

1. **It changes you from the inside out.** It is a deep cleanse that impacts all the cells in the body. PK, taking place over eight days, respects the many layers of the body as well as the time it takes to reach them. This interconnectedness with the dhatus (layers) requires this eight-day cycle.

2. **You will be able to withstand threats and toxins that diminish you.** There is a preventative effect for greater health, as the toxins (*ama*) are removed systematically from the body.

3. **You will experience rejuvenation.** There is a rejuvenation effect on the body and brain as these toxins are reduced in magnitude, thus the natural healing of the body can be re-established. The body can go about its work without all the gunk clogging its capacity to do so.

4. **You will gain clarity.** As the body heals, so does the brain. This impacts our ability to think more clearly.

5. **You will get unstuck.** Emotions become less stuck as well. As the cleanse progresses, it releases emotions, especially toxic ones. The ama is not just at the physical level. And though you can make a note of emotions that are bubbling to the surface, it is best to just witness them and release them in the moment as they appear.

6. **You will release old patterns.** Just as there is cleansing within the cells, there is physical, mental, and emotional cleansing as well. Letting go of old patterns is possible now. That can mean physical habits such as the desire for certain foods and liquids that are only aggravating the body and brain. This can also mean ways of thinking that are not supportive of your well-being. And as you release emotions long stuck within, old patterns of behavior may be altered or no longer present. The subtext of familial patterns can be released. The impact of losing these subtexts can be quite significant for a person. Considering what we are learning about epigenetics, this cleanse could have an impact at the genetic level very easily. And as we release these patterns, we are closer to our true essence, ever closer to our Divine blueprint.

7. **You will find a new equilibrium.** As these old memories/patterns are released, there is an opportunity for a new equilibrium to come into being for you. Choices can present to you that you never would have considered before. You may drop habits that are no longer supportive.

References

Panchakarma

"Ayurveda and Panchakarma: Measuring the Effects of a Holistic Health Intervention," L.A. Conboy, I. Edshteyn, and H. Garivaltis, *Scientific World Journal*. 9: 272–280. *doi:10.1100/tsw.2009.35. Osher Research Center, Harvard Medical School, Boston, MAKripalu, School of Ayurveda, Stockbridge, MA.*

"Identification of Altered Metabolomic Profiles Following a Panchakarma-based Ayurvedic Intervention in Healthy Subjects: The Self-Directed Biological Transformation Initiative"(SBTI). Published February 2016 *Scientific Reports*, volume 6, article number: 32609 (2016) *doi:10.1038/srep32609 Christine Tara Peterson, Joseph Lucas, Lisa St. John-Williams, J. Will Thompson, M. Arthur Moseley, Sheila Patel, Scott N. Peterson, Valencia Porter, Eric E. Schadt, Paul J. Mills, Rudolph E. Tanzi, P. Murali Doraiswamyand Deepak Chopra.*

Medical Conditions

"Rheumatoid Arthritis," *J Ayurveda Integr Med.* 2017 Jan-Mar; 8(1): 42–44. Published online 2017 Mar 14. *doi: 10.1016/j.jaim.2016.10.003.*

Lung Conditions

"Effect of Vasantic Vaman and Other Panchakarma Procedures on Disorders of Various Systems," Mukesh Rawal, K. M. Chudasma,1 R. V. Vyas, 2 and B. P. Parmar3. *Ayu.* 2010 Jul-Sep; 31(3): 319–324. *doi: 10.4103/0974-8520.77160.*

Diabetes

"Comparative Study of Vamana and Virechanakarma in Controlling Blood Sugar Levels in Diabetes Mellitus," Nitin Jindal and Nayan P. Joshi1. Published in *Ayu.* 2013 Jul-Sep; 34(3): 263–269. *doi: 10.4103/0974-8520.123115.*

"Most Inflammatory Conditions and Parkinson's Disorder," Nitin Jindal and Nayan P. Joshi1. Published in *Ayu.* 2013 Jul-Sep; 34(3): 263–269. *doi: 10.4103/0974-8520.123115.*

Acknowledgments

This book was inspired by the many people I have seen in various clinical settings who have willingly shared their suffering, seeking a way out. Their seeking and questions reflected my own journey to find a way beyond the current model of medicine being offered in the West and in most of the rest of the world.

Much gratitude is in my heart for the Divine One leading me to the Joshis and their clinic.

In the world of Ayurveda, Sunil Joshi's own passion for the benefits of Ayurveda and panchakarma (PK) led to the exploration of the benefits of PK for me. I welcomed his wisdom in moving forward with the process and his patience when I would ask about what was unfolding for me. Shalmali Joshi's wisdom supported me during a key time in my journey, for which I am most thankful.

Deepak Chopra's writings, as well as David Frawley's and Vasant Lad's contributions, have also added to the richness of my understanding of Ayurveda and all the other yogas, of which there are eight.

For Pravin, Mukul and his wife, Pritti, and Neetu, as well as the whole staff at the clinic in Nagpur. Their dedication and love created an experience that may be hard to replicate.

For my parents, Matthew and Marie Jose Pentz, who are with the Creator, and who were always supportive of my career as a physician, especially in the years of being a single parent.

For my daughter Danielle and her family, especially Kaynen, for allowing me to be in India for extended periods of time.

For Kathy Franco, MD, my mentor for five years as I trained to become a child, adolescent, and adult psychiatrist, for believing in me along with my intuition and the healer within.

For Carolyn Flynn, whose support in the writing process allowed the fruition of this first endeavor to be birthed into a book.

For the beta readers who read early drafts of the book and cheered me on.

A huge thank you for all who helped with the production of the book: Brenda Knight, editor; Yaddyra Peralta, development editing support; and Robin Miller, for supporting the editing process, as well as the whole Mango Publishing team. This process took place during the COVID 19 crisis, which brought the whole world almost to a full stop, but not this team.

About the Author

For too long, integrative medicine has hovered at the edges of mainstream Western medicine, but what integrative psychiatrist Dr. Judith Eve Pentz brings us *in Cleanse Your Body, Reveal Your Soul* is a map that shows us all how we may integrate these practices into the core of our contemporary lives. She's got the science and the experience, and she's got the soul.

Pentz has practiced as a psychiatrist for thirty years in Albuquerque, New Mexico, where she is on the faculty at the University of New Mexico as an associate professor and attending child, adolescent, and adult psychiatrist. She has often spoken about integrative health, including Ayurvedic healing, in her presentations and written chapters for textbooks published in her field. Since 2018, she has been program director for the Integrative Psychiatry elective in the UNM Department of Psychiatry. Supporting an online curriculum and integrative medicine program started by Andrew Weil from the University of Arizona, she teaches and invites other faculty and community integrative practitioners to share their wisdom in an experiential, didactic manner.

Yet what speaks the loudest as to why she's an authority on the panchakarma cleanse is the manner in which it has profoundly shifted her own life, something she only hoped was possible. She has personally experienced the cleanse and seen the power of it in the significant changes she has instituted in her life, her health, and her career, which continue to unfold.

By training, as a psychiatrist/medical doctor, Pentz has sought ways to help people deeply integrate their own healing at all levels of their being: spiritual, emotional, mental, and physical. In her private practice and her work with children, adolescents, and adults at UNM, she introduces nutrition, meditation, herbs, and nutraceuticals as alternatives to or integrations with Western medicine. In her new work, she shares holistic and healing interventions.

In her work, she has empowered thousands of people to approach their health concerns with a preventative and proactive toolkit. She has an integrative focus in her professional practice, and has a board certification in integrative medicine in addition to child/adolescent and adult psychiatry. She has included interventions for integrative mental health in her practice for over eighteen years.

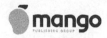

Mango Publishing, established in 2014, publishes an eclectic list of books by diverse authors—both new and established voices—on topics ranging from business, personal growth, women's empowerment, LGBTQ studies, health, and spirituality to history, popular culture, time management, decluttering, lifestyle, mental wellness, aging, and sustainable living. We were recently named 2019 *and* 2020's #1 fastest growing independent publisher by *Publishers Weekly*. Our success is driven by our main goal, which is to publish high quality books that will entertain readers as well as make a positive difference in their lives.

Our readers are our most important resource; we value your input, suggestions, and ideas. We'd love to hear from you—after all, we are publishing books for you!

Please stay in touch with us and follow us at:

Facebook: Mango Publishing
Twitter: @MangoPublishing
Instagram: @MangoPublishing
LinkedIn: Mango Publishing
Pinterest: Mango Publishing

Sign up for our newsletter at www.mangopublishinggroup.com and receive a free book!

Join us on Mango's journey to reinvent publishing, one book at a time.

CPSIA information can be obtained
at www.ICGtesting.com
Printed in the USA
JSHW030420120720
6626JS00004B/10